What You Need to Know about Measles

What You Need to Know about Measles

Patricia Clayton-LeVasseur

Inside Diseases and Disorders

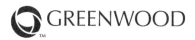

GREENWOOD

An Imprint of ABC-CLIO, LLC

Santa Barbara, California • Denver, Colorado

This book discusses treatments (including types of medication and mental health therapies), diagnostic tests for various symptoms and mental health disorders, and organizations. The authors have made every effort to present accurate and up-to-date information. However, the information in this book is not intended to recommend or endorse particular treatments or organizations, or substitute for the care or medical advice of a qualified health professional, or used to alter any medical therapy without a medical doctor's advice. Specific situations may require specific therapeutic approaches not included in this book. For those reasons, we recommend that readers follow the advice of qualified health care professionals directly involved in their care. Readers who suspect they may have specific medical problems should consult a physician about any suggestions made in this book.

Library of Congress Cataloging-in-Publication Data

Names: Clayton-LeVasseur, Patricia, author.
Title: What you need to know about measles / Patricia Clayton-LeVasseur.
Description: Santa Barbara, California : Greenwood, [2022] | Series: Inside
  diseases and disorders | Includes bibliographical references and index.
Identifiers: LCCN 2022007166 (print) | LCCN 2022007167 (ebook) | ISBN
  9781440875892 (hardcover) | ISBN 9781440875908 (ebook)
Subjects: LCSH: Measles.
Classification: LCC RC168.M4 C53 2022 (print) | LCC RC168.M4 (ebook) |
  DDC 616.9/15—dc23/eng/20220706
LC record available at https://lccn.loc.gov/2022007166
LC ebook record available at https://lccn.loc.gov/2022007167

ISBN: 978-1-4408-7589-2 (print)
         978-1-4408-7590-8 (ebook)

26 25 24 23 22   1 2 3 4 5

This book is also available as an eBook.

Greenwood
An Imprint of ABC-CLIO, LLC

ABC-CLIO, LLC
147 Castilian Drive
Santa Barbara, California 93117
www.abc-clio.com

This book is printed on acid-free paper ∞

Manufactured in the United States of America

*This book is dedicated to my
wonderful husband, Dr. James LeVasseur.
I am grateful that I can share my life with someone
who helps me appreciate the present and
remain hopeful for the future.*

Contents

CHAPTER 8
Prevention *81*

CHAPTER 9
Issues and Controversies *99*

CHAPTER 10
Current Research and Future Directions *119*

Series Foreword

Disease is as old as humanity itself, and it has been the leading cause of death and disability throughout history. From the Black Death in the Middle Ages to smallpox outbreaks among Native Americans to the modern-day epidemics of diabetes and heart disease, humans have lived with—and died from—all manner of ailments, whether caused by infectious agents, environmental and lifestyle factors, or genetic abnormalities. The field of medicine has been driven forward by our desire to combat and prevent disease and to improve the lives of those living with debilitating disorders. And while we have made great strides forward, particularly in the last 100 years, it is doubtful that mankind will ever be completely free of the burden of disease.

Greenwood's Inside Diseases and Disorders series examines some of the key diseases and disorders, both physical and psychological, affecting the world today. Some (such as diabetes, cardiovascular disease, and attention-deficit hyperactivity disorder) have been selected because of their prominence within modern America. Others (such as Ebola, celiac disease, and autism) have been chosen because they are often discussed in the media and, in some cases, are controversial or the subject of scientific or cultural debate.

Because this series covers so many different diseases and disorders, we have striven to create uniformity across all books. To maximize clarity and consistency, each book in the series follows the same format. Each begins with a collection of frequently asked questions about the disease or disorder, followed by clear, concise answers. Chapter 1 provides a general introduction to the disease or disorder, including statistical information such as prevalence rates and demographic trends. The history of the disease or disorder, including how our understanding of it has evolved over time, is addressed in chapter 2. Chapter 3 examines causes and risk factors, whether genetic, microbial, or environmental, while chapter 4 discusses signs and symptoms. Chapter 5 covers the issues of diagnosis (and misdiagnosis), treatment, and management (whether with drugs, medical procedures, or lifestyle changes). How such treatment, or the lack thereof, affects a patient's long-term prognosis, as well as the risk of complications, are the subject of chapter 6. Chapter 7 explores the disease or disorder's effects on the friends and family of a patient—a dimension often overlooked in discussions of physical and psychological ailments. Chapter 8 discusses prevention strategies, while chapter 9 explores key issues or controversies, whether medical or sociocultural. Finally, chapter 10 profiles cutting-edge research and speculates on how things might change in the next few decades.

Each volume also features five fictional case studies to illustrate different aspects of the book's subject matter, highlighting key concepts and themes that have been explored throughout the text. The reader will also find a glossary of terms and a collection of print and electronic resources for additional information and further study.

As a final caveat, please be aware that the information presented in these books is no substitute for consultation with a licensed health-care professional. These books do not claim to provide medical advice or guidance.

Acknowledgments

To my dedicated parents, William and Ann Clayton, you provided support and encouragement when I doubted myself. Thank you for your daily demonstration of God's love.

To Nathan, Courtney, and Chelsea, you always make me smile! Thank you for your support in this journey.

To my friend Dr. Angela Wilder, you have been my "sister" for over forty years. I am thankful for your willingness to always be available for conversation and advice.

Introduction

Human history indicates a presence of measles in the ninth century by Muhammad ibn Zakariya al-Razi (865–925 CE), or Rhazes, a Persian doctor who differentiated smallpox and measles. Rhazes wrote of a disease that appeared when herd animals such as goats, sheep, and cattle were domesticated. During this time, humans were exposed to animal-specific viruses because they lived among these animals, and the virus moved from animal to human hosts. One of the viruses of long standing has been the rinderpest virus found in cattle, also known as cattle's measles. The rinderpest virus eventually evolved into today's measles virus, which spread exponentially from 2016 to 2019 and claimed the lives of over 207,500 people worldwide.

Measles is an aerosolized virus that originates in an infected person's saliva and respiratory secretions and is then expelled into the air by coughing, sneezing, talking, or even breathing. Scientists at the Centers for Disease Control and Prevention (CDC) report that the virus expelled into the air from an infectious person can remain infectious on hard surfaces for up to two hours. Anyone who comes into contact with these surfaces and then touches their nose, mouth, or eyes can become infected. Unvaccinated people, anyone with a compromised immune system, and individuals residing in developing countries with inadequate vaccination programs are at the highest risk of becoming infected with measles and developing severe complications resulting from the disease.

Measles, or rubeola, is a highly contagious virus. It is so infectious that 90 percent of unvaccinated people exposed to this virus will become infected. Symptoms usually develop ten to twelve days after exposure and last approximately two weeks. The classic symptoms include a cough, coryza (runny nose), and conjunctivitis (inflamed eyes); a fever accompanies the vague symptoms. Odd bluish-white spots appear inside a person's mouth and are called *Koplik's spots*, after Dr. Henry Koplik (1858–1927).

They are considered a definitive symptom of measles and present before the hallmark maculopapular rash (a flat, reddened area on the skin). The classic measles rash begins on the skin along the hairline and face before it spreads downward and all over the body. Recognizing these spots is an early clue that the person has measles and should be isolated.

Measles can be spread to others four days before the rash's appearance and lasts one to two weeks. The contagious person must be isolated in the early stages of the illness to prevent measles spread. Anyone who had been in contact with the person during the days just before the rash appeared must be informed of possible exposure. Measles is a notifiable disease in many nations, including the United States, the United Kingdom, Australia, and many European countries. Notifiable diseases require that confirmed cases be reported to government authorities. Although all countries should consider measles a notifiable disease, some developing countries do not have the infrastructure to support this endeavor. The public health agencies in all countries assist in surveillance, which triggers a search for additional cases, usually from schools or health-care providers. Measles primarily affects the school-aged population, and, historically, this group has difficulty complying with habits that prevent the spread of illness, such as hand hygiene.

The diagnosis of measles is dependent on the signs and symptoms of the person. These symptoms often resolve within two to three weeks without additional treatment, such as antibiotics or antiviral medication. Common complications occur in one out of ten measles cases and can include ear infections and diarrhea. Severe complications, including pneumonia and encephalitis, are rare but tend to affect mostly young children under five years of age. According to the CDC, up to three out of 1,000 children will die from neurological or respiratory complications from measles.

The two-dose combined measles, mumps, and rubella (MMR) vaccine offers 97 percent protection against measles. The World Health Organization (WHO) considers the vaccine a safe and inexpensive method to prevent measles. Most people who receive it do not have any complications, and it is much safer than getting the naturally occurring measles virus. Some people are opposed to vaccines. Anti-vaxxers believe that vaccinations are unsafe, a form of genocidal weapon, or used for surveillance. They also believe that a requirement of universal vaccination is an infringement on their human rights. In 2021, *Men's Health* published an article titled "The Golden Age of Junk Science" by Timothy Caulfield that exposes science misinformation and the prevalence of unsubstantiated "research" that has become a driving force in the general public's opinions on medical matters. The pervasive use of social media has skewed the legitimacy of scientific research that is valid and reliable.

Some anti-vaccination organizations argue that there is a link between vaccinations and autism, allegedly found by the English doctor Andrew Wakefield and his colleagues. Their study was published in the medical journal *The Lancet* in 1998, but it was later redacted because the researchers had falsified the results and engaged in unethical practices. There is no scientific link between the MMR vaccine and autism, but some people cling to the unsupported belief that the MMR vaccine can result in autism. Their doubt of scientific reasoning has resulted in children and adults who are not vaccinated.

A global resurgence of measles is spreading at present. The *Global Measles and Rubella Strategic Plan, 2012–2020* attempted to vaccinate 90 percent of the children worldwide with the MMR vaccine, but the initiative was unsuccessful due to the lack of unified government support and inequalities of vaccine programs. Now a new barrier is preventing effective vaccination, the coronavirus (COVID-19). Due to the pandemic, the primary focus has shifted from childhood vaccinations to the new FDA-approved COVID-19 vaccines. The testing, production, and administration of the vaccines for COVID-19 is taxing the already strained global health-care systems. The future is primed for a measles resurrection, which will be costly for the world's health-care infrastructure and deadly for many.

Essential Questions

1. CAN THE MEASLES, MUMPS, AND RUBELLA (MMR) VACCINE CAUSE MEASLES?

The measles, mumps, and rubella (MMR) vaccine is an attenuated (weak) form of the measles, mumps, and rubella viruses. Measles present with a fever, rash, cough, coryza (runny nose), and conjunctivitis (inflamed eyes). Mumps cause a fever, headache, lethargy (tiredness), muscle aches, and swollen glands. The symptoms of rubella also cause a fever, rash, and headache. The person receiving the vaccine may develop some of the symptoms of one or more of these viruses: However, the signs and symptoms are much milder than from the naturally acquired diseases. When a person develops symptoms after receiving the MMR vaccine, it is deemed an adverse reaction to receiving the vaccine. The person is not diagnosed with having the naturally occurring measles, mumps, or rubella.

2. WHY DO SOME PARENTS CHOOSE NOT TO VACCINATE THEIR CHILDREN?

The most common reason parents choose not to vaccinate their children is the fear that the vaccine will cause autistic or Asperger's spectrum disorder, commonly called *autism*. Autism affects the brain and the person's ability to communicate and interact with others. The exact cause is unknown but has been linked to anatomical differences and exposure to toxic substances. Multiple studies support the conclusion that there is no link between autism and receiving the MMR vaccine. In 2013, an autism research study funded by the Centers for Disease Control and Prevention (CDC) evaluated the process of how a child's immune system produces antigens (disease-fighting antibodies) between children who have been diagnosed with autism spectrum disorder (ASD) and those who did not have this disability. The study concluded that the antigens were the same for both populations. A 2015 study published in the *Journal of American Medical Association* (JAMA) evaluated the link between autism and the MMR vaccine. The study assessed 95,727 children; 1,929 were considered high-risk children with a genetic predisposition to autism because an older sibling had been diagnosed with this disability. The large retrospective study concluded that receiving the MMR vaccine did not increase the risk of developing autism, even if the child had an older sibling with autism.

3. IN WHAT PART OF THE WORLD IS MEASLES A COMMON DISEASE?

Measles is common in many developing countries, including Ukraine, Madagascar, India, Pakistan, the Philippines, Yemen, and Brazil. According to the World Health Organization (WHO), Madagascar recorded more than 69,000 cases and 1,200 deaths in 2018; this is the most massive and devastating measles outbreak for the island. Africa and Asia are also severely affected, as approximately seven million people in these two continents have been affected by measles. The predominance of measles deaths has been shown to occur in countries with weak health-care infrastructure and low per capita incomes, as reported by the WHO in 2019.

4. WHAT IS THE FIRST SIGN OF MEASLES?

The measles virus incubates for the first ten to fourteen days after exposure, during which time there are no signs or symptoms of measles. The early signs and symptoms are flu-like and include general malaise and poor appetite. The three hallmark symptoms are a cough, conjunctivitis, and coryza. The person will have an abnormally high fever (104 degrees Fahrenheit to 105 degrees Fahrenheit). A rash will appear near the hairline on the face and spread down the entire body. The rash consists of small red spots that are numerous and closely spaced. Places inside the mouth appear as white areas with a bluish-white center and red background; these are called *Koplik's spots.*

5. CAN CHILDREN GET MEASLES EVEN IF THEY ARE VACCINATED?

It is rare for a vaccinated child to get measles after the MMR vaccination. The MMR is a two-dose vaccination series that safely protects children from measles, mumps, and rubella. The first dose of the MMR vaccine is administered between the ages of twelve months and fifteen months. This vaccination provides a protection rate of 95 percent. The second dose is administered between the ages of four and six years, before the child attends a day care facility or school. The second dose of the MMR vaccine provides a protection rate of 97 percent. The risk of exposure to measles increases if the child is traveling abroad, so the first and second doses may be administered earlier than customarily scheduled to offset that risk. According to the CDC, children who get two doses of measles vaccine have less than a 3 percent chance of getting measles.

6. DOES THE MEASLES VACCINE PROVIDE LIFELONG PROTECTION?

The MMR vaccine is widely accepted as a safe and effective method of protecting the general public with normal immune systems from measles, mumps, and rubella. Persons in the United States who have received the two-dose MMR vaccine are considered protected for life; no booster is needed under normal circumstances. Nevertheless, many health-care agencies support the practice of having a third, or booster, vaccination during measles outbreaks. This practice is especially true for health-care providers, elderly persons, and those with an impaired immune response.

7. CAN A CHILD LESS THAN ONE YEAR OF AGE RECEIVE THE MEASLES VACCINE?

The CDC recommends that children receive their first MMR vaccination between twelve months and fifteen months of age. This timeline is based on the naturally acquired maternal antibodies that protect the child until they are a year old, meaning that the vaccination would be ineffective before this time. Children who are less than one year of age and will be traveling abroad can receive the first MMR vaccine around six months of age prior to travel. This is especially important if the travel is planned for countries with a current outbreak. The second dose can follow the regular inoculation schedule and be administered between twelve months and fifteen months. The CDC recommends a third dose between the ages of four and six for children who have received a vaccination earlier than typically scheduled. If the child is traveling to a country currently experiencing a measles outbreak, a booster shot can be administered four weeks after the initial dose. It is recommended that parents with infants and children contact their health-care provider and discuss their children's vaccination schedule.

8. CAN A VACCINATED PERSON SPREAD MEASLES?

A child or adult who has only received one dose of the MMR vaccination series has a minimal probability of becoming infected with the measles virus. The first dose provides a 95 percent protection rate against contracting measles. A child or adult who receives the second dose of the MMR has a 97 percent protection rate and is deemed fully protected from measles. This means that the person cannot spread measles to another person, even though some research suggests that a vaccinated person has less than a 3 percent chance of spreading the virus to a vulnerable person. This would include unvaccinated children and adults, infants less than six months of age, and those diagnosed with a disease that renders them immunocompromised. There is only a slight possibility that a vaccinated person can spread measles due to the pathophysiological process that occurs when the person is vaccinated. The vaccine initiates a "seek and destroy mission" when a vaccinated person is exposed to the virus and will attach itself to and kill the measles virus, rendering it no longer able to replicate within the person's body.

9. WHAT ARE THE COMMON SIDE EFFECTS OF THE MEASLES VACCINE?

The MMR vaccine is considered much safer than the naturally occurring viruses, even though some individuals may develop a mild reaction. The MMR vaccine's most common side effects are fever, slight rash, and pain at the injection site. The MMR vaccine has been associated with febrile seizures in infants in some cases. This form of seizure risk increases with age and is temporary. The CDC reports that 4 out of 10,000 children who receive the vaccine between the ages of twelve and twenty-four months will have a fever and subsequently have a febrile seizure approximately seven days after the immunization. Children vaccinated between two and seven years of age have a one in 4,000 risk of having a febrile seizure. Adults have relatively no risk of febrile seizures.

10. CAN MEASLES KILL YOU?

In 1963, before the development of the MMR vaccine, the worldwide rate of death from measles each year was 2.6 million people. This number has decreased substantially with numerous vaccination campaigns. Today, one out of every 1,000 children who contract measles will die from respiratory or neurological complications. The most common life-threatening side effect is pneumonia, which requires aggressive treatment and hospitalization.

1

What Is Measles?

Measles is a highly contagious virus that can be effortlessly transmitted by direct or indirect routes, especially when an infected person sneezes or coughs; the virus is spread to others nearby. The infection can also be spread by kissing or sharing the same glass or eating utensils. The ability of the virus to be transmitted before any symptoms appear is of great concern.

The signs and symptoms of measles appear ten days after exposure, during which time the person is considered contagious and can infect others. The hallmark signs of measles are a rash, cough, runny nose, and inflammation of the eyes. Most people will also have a fever. The symptoms generally only require treatment with over-the-counter medications. However, in some conditions, complications from the disease can range from mild to life-threatening. Diarrhea, vomiting, and respiratory difficulties are among the most common mild complications, while the onset of pneumonia is the most common cause of mortality.

Viral infection of measles is prevented through the measles, mumps, and rubella (MMR) two-dose vaccination series or natural immunity. With the MMR vaccines, a person will attain 97 percent protection. Innate immunity resulting from having been infected with measles offers 100 percent lifetime protection. Measles was believed to have been eradicated in the United States in 2000 as a notifiable disease; however, outbreaks are trending today due to increased international travel and because there are parents (anti-vaxxers) who choose not to vaccinate their children due to the (scientifically debunked) belief that vaccines cause other serious health problems or for philosophical or religious reasons.

THE RUBEOLA VIRUS

The rubeola virus, or measles, belongs to the viral family *Paramyxoviridae*. This viral family includes morbillivirus in dolphins and porpoises, the canine distemper virus in dogs, and the rinderpest virus (RPV) found in cattle. Scientist have linked the virus to 600 BCE, during the period that coincides with the emergence of large human settlements living among domesticated cattle. Measles mimicked the rinderpest virus's genetics and is believed by medical historians to have diverged from rinderpest due to humans living among the cattle. Divergence is the process by which a virus changes from one genetic strain into a different genetic structure, thus allowing the virus to mutate from animals to humans.

The mutation timeline was determined through molecular clock analysis, a scientific method of aging prehistoric biomolecules, and by examining various viruses' genetic sequences. The genetic sequences of the rubeola and rinderpest viruses came from a publicly available repository of all known nucleotide sequences, known as the GenBank. Scientists used the genetic sequences of the viruses to calculate their mutation rates to predict when the genetic structures of measles evolved from a bovine virus to become a separate entity in human hosts.

Rubeola versus Rubella

Over twenty different measles strains originate from the morbillivirus and rinderpest viruses, but all measles viruses have a specific serotype. There are two primary forms: rubeola and rubella. Rubella is also known as German measles or three-day measles. This form is milder, and the symptoms are similar to rubeola. The initial symptoms are flu-like and include fatigue, low-grade fever, headache, and irritated eyes. Studies have shown that approximately 50 percent of confirmed rubella cases have no symptoms at all and resolve in a few days without medical intervention. German measles also presents with a rash, but it is usually light pink and may not itch or be painful. Patients are contagious several days before the outbreak and seven days after the rash dissipates, very much like rubeola.

The most severe complication occurs during pregnancy, when the virus spreads from an infected pregnant woman to her unborn child through the bloodstream. This situation is of particular concern because the fetus may develop congenital rubella, resulting in myriad congenital disabilities. The most common of these are cataracts, heart defects, hearing loss, and learning disabilities. The mother who contracts rubella during the first trimester has increased risk of congenital disabilities in the fetus. Having a miscarriage or stillbirth may also be a tragic complication of the virus. The prevention of rubella is simple with the MMR vaccine. This vaccine contains the attenuated (weak) rubella and rubeola viruses and effectively protects children and adults from contracting the illnesses.

Herd Immunity

People infected with measles retain a lifelong immunity. A constant supply of susceptible individuals is required for the disease to maintain virality. Herd immunity postulates that when a large portion of the general population is immune to the disease through antibodies from the infection or a vaccine, it provides passive protection for the unvaccinated. This dynamic suggests that eradicating the virus is possible if the susceptible population becomes too small for continuous transmission. This phenomenon has been seen in communities, geographic areas, and countries with consistent vaccinations.

For herd immunity to protect the unvaccinated people, 95 percent of the population worldwide would either have immunity from naturally occurring measles or have received the two-dose MMR vaccine. This means that every person of every age group, geographical area, and cultural subgroup would be considered protected from measles. Many in the health-care community believe that this is a difficult, if not impossible, goal to achieve. However, a few countries with mandatory vaccinations have achieved herd immunity for measles. According to the World Health Organization (WHO), Germany and Serbia have strict rules on the vaccination of all preschool- and school-aged children and have achieved herd immunity. However, both countries still have isolated outbreaks.

MEASLES IS A HIGHLY CONTAGIOUS INFECTION

Measles cannot survive or reproduce without a host. The virus reproduces by attaching itself to a host cell and injecting its genetic material into it. The virus reprograms the host cells to make new viral cells and continues to reproduce until the cell dies. When measles enters a host's body, it initiates its attack in the respiratory system. It essentially establishes itself in the mucosal membranes of the nose and throat in the infected child or adult. Once the virus has established a colony in the respiratory system, measles expands its environment and spreads to the lymphatic and nervous systems, blood vessels, and the eyes.

A person is contagious for several days before symptoms develop a trait that makes it difficult to arrest the spread of measles. The virus may take anywhere from seven to twenty-one days to become established in the body, but symptoms will appear in approximately ten days. Close proximity to a contagious person, such as living in the same house or dormitory or being in an enclosed area, such as a plane or a classroom, increases the risk of contracting the infection. A reddish-brown rash that typically starts on the face and then spreads downward until it covers the entire body is a telltale sign of measles's onset. A person is considered contagious for four days before presenting a rash and four to five days after the rash disappears. During this infectious period, 90 percent of those in close contact with the infected person will become infected themselves (unless they have already had measles or have been vaccinated) through direct contact or from touching a contaminated object or surface.

THOSE AT GREATEST RISK

Newborns are incredibly vulnerable to measles, especially since they are too young to receive the MMR vaccine. A newborn's immune system is immature and unable to generate a protective immunological response to the vaccination. Having the MMR vaccine earlier than one year of age increases the risk of severe complications such as pneumonia. Antibodies transferred from the pregnant mother offer some protection but not 100 percent immunity. The Centers for Disease Control and Prevention (CDC) recommends using caution with infants in areas with a current outbreak and limiting public exposure.

Children are the most vulnerable population to contracting measles, especially those under five years of age. The WHO published a report on child mortality in 2019 and listed measles in the top five causes of death for children worldwide. Pneumonia is the most common cause of death for children with measles. The CDC (2019) reported 500,000 pneumonia cases among children in the United States, of which 48,000 required hospitalizations and 450 died. The Infectious Diseases Society of America (2015) suggests that approximately nine million children are highly susceptible to getting measles because they are unvaccinated or undervaccinated. Unvaccinated or undervaccinated children (infants to eighteen-year-olds) are the age group who are the most prone to measles.

Unfortunately, some children and adults cannot receive the MMR vaccine due to certain diseases or being immunocompromised. A person diagnosed with cancer and undergoing chemotherapy or high-dose steroids should not get inoculated. The MMR vaccine is a live attenuated (weakened) strain of measles, and the person would not have the ability to develop antibodies; instead, they could develop measles with dangerous complications. Specific allergies also prohibit some from getting inoculated due to anaphylactic shock (severe allergic reaction).

Others are at risk due to being undervaccinated, or partially vaccinated. Either they did not receive the second dose of MMR or were exposed between the first and second doses. Some also fail to develop full immunity to measles, even with the two doses given at the recommended ages. Approximately 3 percent of the general public will not serum convert and produce antibodies. A person would not be aware of this factor until after being exposed to the virus and becoming symptomatic. Partially vaccinated individuals or those who do not serum convert can get measles, a condition known as modified measles, which fortunately is usually less severe and contagious.

Another at-risk group is those who received a vaccine between the years 1963 and 1967. Vaccines given during this period may have contained an inactive (killed) virus, which offers no protection against measles. Most adults are unaware of the ineffectiveness of the vaccine and consider themselves entirely immune. It is only after measles symptoms develop that they will seek advice on their immunity status. Atypical measles symptoms are more severe and generally begin with fever and headache. The measles rash will start on the wrists or ankles with minimal or no facial rash.

Another risk factor is vitamin A deficiency. Vitamin A does not prevent measles infection, but it can mitigate symptoms and severe complications. International travel to countries currently experiencing a measles outbreak increases the risk for exposure and becoming infected. Some physicians recommend receiving an MMR booster shot before leaving the United States, especially for children or the elderly.

The most critical risk factors for measles infection are being unvaccinated or undervaccinated. The WHO, the CDC, and the American Academy of Pediatrics (AAP) all support the practice of two-dose MMR vaccination as the only secure method to protect against measles.

SIGNS AND SYMPTOMS OF MEASLES

Measles follow a reasonably predictable symptomatic timeline (see below diagram). The virus sheds from the nasopharynx area of an infected person's mouth and throat until three to four days after the rash appears, known as the prodromal period. The incubation period extends from the

Timeline	Symptoms
Onset	Sudden fever and malaise
Days 1–2	Coryza, conjunctivitis, and cough
Days 3–4	Koplik's spots
Days 10–14	Body rash
Day 14	Symptoms begin to resolve

point of exposure to prodrome, which in the case of measles, is an average of ten days before the first symptoms appear. During this incubation period, the child may be irritable and lethargic. The child may withdraw or complain of not feeling well and cry for no apparent reason. The sudden onset of fever will follow, ranging from mild (99 degrees Fahrenheit to 101 degrees Fahrenheit) to high enough to cause seizures (103 degrees Fahrenheit to 104 degrees Fahrenheit). The fever lasts from four to five days and often spikes in the evening. Around twenty-four hours after the fever, three classic cold symptoms begin: a cough, coryza (runny nose), and conjunctivitis (inflamed eyes). The afflicted child is not hungry or only eats small amounts and stops consistent water drinking, resulting in mild dehydration. Sunlight may cause the child to squint because of photophobia (sensitivity to light).

A maculopapular rash will appear along the hairline, forehead, and behind the earlobes approximately ten to fourteen days after exposure. This rash will then travel to the neck and spread across the body over the next few days. Infants and children may develop diarrhea and generalized lymphadenopathy (enlargement of the lymph glands). The upper-body rash often appears to merge into one sizable reddened area and is painful and itchy. The outbreak rash is maculopapular (flat and red), blanching with pressure in its initial presentation, then it gradually morphs into brownish spots until it disappears, around day six.

Although measles is predominantly a childhood illness, adults can also get the disease. Adults will present with the same symptoms as children, fever, cough, coryza, and conjunctivitis. However, adults often experience more severe symptoms, and respiratory complications often result in pneumonia.

COMPLICATIONS OF MEASLES

Complications from measles range from mild to severe. The CDC (2015) reports that around 30 percent of confirmed measles cases in the United

States will have one or more complications. Respiratory difficulties are the most common, resulting in laryngitis, bronchitis, and pneumonia. The infection produces thick, tenacious sputum and a deficiency in oxygen levels, a condition that promotes the onset of pneumonia. Pneumonia is an infection in the lungs that inhibits normal lung function, causing shortness of breath and chest pain when breathing. This infection reduces the lung's ability to exchange oxygen and carbon dioxide. Pneumonia is the most common complication of measles for children and adults. Usually, an adult with pneumonia from measles will require hospitalization and in some cases mechanical ventilation. Approximately one in four adults over the age of twenty will be hospitalized, and one to two per thousand will die.

Other mild to moderate complications include diarrhea and vomiting, which are usually short term. Although uncomfortable, they are not life-threatening. However, if they are severe or persistent, they can result in dehydration. Severe dehydration may cause kidney damage. Anyone with diarrhea or vomiting should seek medical care and be encouraged to increase their fluid intake.

Conjunctivitis is a mild but annoying complication of measles. Eye infections are often associated with conjunctivitis, but most cases respond well to antibiotic eye drops. Rarely, conjunctivitis can cause permanent nerve damage, constant squinting, permanent visual deficits, and vision loss, although this is not common. Severe complications are discussed in detail in chapter 4.

A person with measles will usually have a fever. Fevers higher than 104 degrees Fahrenheit may result in febrile seizures or convulsions, sometimes lasting for several minutes. Febrile seizures are frequent in children but, fortunately, usually transient.

Other complications from measles are more severe. Brain inflammation, known as encephalitis, occurs in one out of every thousand people with measles. The most common complaints resulting from encephalitis are headaches and confusion. Encephalitis may result in permanent neurological deficits or even death. The patient may hallucinate and develop seizures as the condition progresses. Long term, the patient may have cognitive deficits, blindness, or hearing loss.

Hepatitis or liver complications can occur due to the administration of antibiotics and antiviral medications. Thrombocytopenia is another potential complication in which the platelet count is low, reducing the blood's ability to form a clot. Measles may also cause cardiac dysthymias (irregular beating of the heart), resulting in decreased blood flow to vital organs or myocardial infarction (damage to the cardiac muscle). Pregnant women who contract measles are at higher risk for premature labor, low infant birth weight, and even maternal death.

MORTALITY OF MEASLES

Deaths from measles have declined by 84 percent worldwide from 2010 to 2016; even so, deaths still occur. Before the invention of a measles vaccine, approximately 500,000 cases were documented in the United States, and 500 of those cases resulted in death. The WHO estimates that more than 140,000 deaths from measles occur annually, mostly among children under age five.

Alarmingly, more than twenty million infants worldwide are unvaccinated, and measles continues to be a significant factor in infant mortality such that even today, the battle to eradicate this virus continues. Evidence suggests that girls have a higher mortality rate than boys diagnosed with measles, which is not the case for most infectious diseases. School-aged children of both sexes have an increased susceptibility to measles in late winter and early spring. This seasonal outbreak is associated with attending school and school-related activities. Tropical areas report most epidemics during the rainy season, when the general population is confined to indoor activities.

The WHO has declared that measles could be eradicated in most of the world by utilizing a global vaccination plan. This plan should focus on providing vaccinations to underdeveloped countries with minimal to no vaccination programs. The barriers to the project include the financial cost of the human resources to administer the vaccines, not necessarily the actual cost of the vaccine, which is less than two dollars. Additionally, many developing countries have a weak infrastructure for health care. Without a stable health-care distribution plan, providing the vaccines is unreliable. Further, countries must address parental resistance to vaccinating children.

DIAGNOSIS AND TREATMENT

The diagnosis of measles is dependent on the signs and symptoms of the person. Physicians in the United States receive extensive education on recognizing infectious diseases, including measles. The diagnosis of measles depends on the child or adult having all of the following symptoms: fever, rash, cough, conjunctivitis, and coryza. Although a blood test can confirm the diagnosis, it is rarely used because most physicians diagnose measles based on the symptoms and presentation of the hallmark rash.

There is no definitive care plan for measles; most doctors endorse plenty of fluids, rest, and limited exposure to the general public. Although the infected person may not require prescriptions, measles will frequently result in lethargy, intense pain, itching from the rash, and fever. These symptoms often resolve within two to three weeks without additional treatment, such as antibiotics or antiviral medication.

Infected people should isolate themselves during the contagious period, even though being separated from friends is often difficult for children and teenagers; the isolation may produce anger or depression. Parents and health-care providers must inform the school system that the child attends so that notifications can be sent to the parents of the other children who may have been exposed. The child cannot return to school for at least five days after the rash appears or when free of a fever for forty-eight hours. Adults must also isolate themselves during the infectious period; they sometimes miss several weeks of work and may incur significant financial difficulties. Measles is considered a notifiable disease in the United States. Any incidence of the disease must be promptly reported to the local health-care department.

AN ENDEMIC DISEASE

The word *endemic* stems from the Greek word *endemos*, which consists of two words, "en," meaning "in," and "demos," meaning "people or population." The literal translation, according to *Merriam-Webster*, is "in the population." An endemic disease occurs permanently in a geographic region or population at a consistent baseline without external influence. Malaria is endemic in many areas of Africa. Hepatitis B is an endemic disease worldwide, and the infection rates continue to rise in many countries. In the United States, the vaccine for the hepatitis B virus (HBV) is part of the standardized childhood immunization schedule.

There are two types of endemic diseases: holoendemic and hyperendemic. A *holoendemic* disease affects every person within a geographical area; ocular trachoma is an eye infection from the bacteria *Chlamydia trachomatis* and is prevalent in the Middle East, North Africa, and sub-Saharan Africa. With this disease, both eyes will have itching and scaling on the inner surface of the eyes. The bacterial infection responds quickly to antibiotics if treatment begins in the early stages, but the spread of this infection makes it the leading cause of preventable blindness worldwide.

Hyperendemic diseases are defined as having high and continuous incidence; they affect all ages and genders alike and are not influenced by the different seasons. One example of a hyperendemic disease is dengue hemorrhagic fever. This illness is an acute febrile (fever-related) disease spread by mosquitos. Global concern is growing, as cases are increasing from globalization patterns and climate changes. Approximately fifty million people are infected by dengue fever annually worldwide. The WHO considers dengue fever a controllable disease through governing or eradicating the *Aedes* mosquito that carries the highly contagious virus. Still, this goal is unachievable without assistance from local government agencies and public health officials controlling the *Aedes* mosquito.

Measles is no longer an endemic disease in North, Central, and South America. Currently, Venezuela and Brazil have reestablished measles as an endemic disease. The top five countries with the highest number of vaccinated children include Pakistan, Yemen, Tanzania, India, and Nigeria. In Pakistan, measles has been endemic for several years and accounts for 65 percent of the total measles burden for the Eastern Mediterranean region. The Democratic Republic of the Congo, South Africa, and Afghanistan all report measles as endemic.

The last endemic measles diagnosis for North and South America was in 2002. Although measles was considered eradicated on these continents, outbreaks still occur in isolated geographical areas where unvaccinated people congregate. International travelers are additionally at increased risk of contracting measles during trips to countries where vaccinations are not prevalent. Once contagious, a person can expose approximately 90 percent of unvaccinated people through direct or indirect contact (WHO, 2019).

An epidemic differs from an endemic. An *epidemic* describes an illness as a sudden and severe outbreak within a geographical area or population, as seen with AIDS in Africa. A *pandemic* is a disease that is so virulent that it affects states, continents, or the entire world. A prime example of a pandemic is COVID-19. This novel virus has infected over 219 million people globally and explicitly affects the elderly population. However, new variant strains of the virus appear to be nondiscriminatory and more infectious. The WHO reports over 4.5 million people have died from COVID-19 worldwide. The United States will have over 963,000 deaths recorded by March 2022 based on the CDC's statistics.

A NOTIFIABLE DISEASE

Notifiable diseases are also termed reportable because they are considered essential to the health and well-being of the general population, and such reports are required by law to be conveyed to government authorities. Notification is needed for monitoring and preventing potential outbreaks. Examples of such diseases include gonorrhea, rubeola (measles), pertussis (whooping cough), chickenpox, and influenza, to name a few. Notification of these diseases allows government and health-care agencies to collect statistical data and enables public health officials to predict disease trends and track current outbreaks. The goal of the regulatory agencies is to curb future occurrences.

Surveillance for certain diseases and illnesses is conducted by local, national, and international sources on a continual basis. Local public health officials monitor their regional population for specific diagnoses. At the federal level, the CDC collects and maintains disease statistics. The WHO is the premier international organization that oversees the global status of infections and sicknesses.

Reporting Process

Reporting a notifiable disease in the United States is the obligation of all health-care providers and facilities to local regulatory agencies. Other diseases must be notified directly to the CDC. The protocol for identifying and reporting notifiable conditions is updated yearly by the CDC. The reporting system categorizes diseases into three notification timelines: (1) immediate notification and extremely urgent, (2) immediate notification and urgent, and (3) routinely notifiable. Immediately notifiable and extremely urgent conditions require health-care agencies to call the CDC's Emergency Operations Center within four hours of a case meeting this criterion. Eight diseases meet the standards of immediate notification and extremely urgent: anthrax (not naturally occurring), botulism plague, paralytic poliomyelitis, SARS-associated coronavirus, smallpox, tularemia, and viral hemorrhagic fevers. Viral hemorrhagic fevers include Ebola and yellow fever. These eight conditions have a high mortality rate and carry the potential to initiate an epidemic or pandemic.

Anthrax (naturally occurring), brucellosis, diphtheria, influenza A virus, measles, polio, rabies, and rubella meet the definition of immediate notification and urgent. Conditions meeting this criterion must be called in to the Emergency Operations Center within twenty-four hours of presentation and have an electronic case notification submitted to public health officials. Numerous conditions are routinely notifiable to the CDC: cancer, gonorrhea, hepatitis, human immunodeficiency virus (HIV), and Lyme disease are among this group. Notifications for these conditions are sent during prescheduled reporting cycles to the CDC.

Measles has been a notifiable disease since 1912 in the United States. All health-care providers and laboratories have been required to report this diagnosis as an immediate notification in the urgent category. The goal of reporting is to quickly identify everyone who has been exposed to measles, prevent the spread of measles, and categorize populations of unvaccinated children and adults. The legal reporting requirements begin with health-care providers, facilities, and laboratories with a patient or specimen that meets or presents as a potential measles diagnosis.

Once notified by the CDC, local public health jurisdictions, such as health departments, begin investigating all confirmed and probable cases. The public health authorities mandate that any person with an actual diagnosis of measles must isolate for a minimum of four days after the onset of the rash. Susceptible contacts are located and informed of possible exposure and instructed to follow-up with their health-care provider. Assistance by public health officials is offered to businesses and schools where the infected individual may have visited. Laboratories must also submit any specimens with a positive result within two business days to the public health laboratories for further testing. Surveillance by public health officials begins for additional cases.

Case Definition

The clinical case definition for measles must meet the following characteristics: (1) generalized rash that lasts for more than three days, (2) fever that is greater than 101 degrees Fahrenheit, and (3) one or more of the following: cough, coryza, and conjunctivitis. Upon diagnosis, a routine investigation begins by reviewing the medical history, international travel, physical presentation, and potential exposure period of between seven and twenty-one days before the onset of a rash. The most crucial health history information to include is the immunization records. If needed, a blood test can confirm measles antibodies for vaccinated individuals. Testing is usually not advised for a person who does not exhibit the clinical case definition criteria or is recently immunized. All situations require clinical judgment from the health-care provider and public health personnel. The individuals who meet the clinical case definition will have blood drawn, urine collected, and respiratory specimens obtained.

The next step with notifiable conditions is to identify the potential sources of measles. This process includes the activities of the person being evaluated, particularly during the peak exposure period between seven and twenty-one days before the onset of a rash. Additional resources are needed to identify indoor activities or group activities, such as theaters, parties, and travel, as these activities could result in exposure to many people. Health-care providers or public health officials will contact all known persons, especially those who have developed a rash, traveled (within or outside the United States), or interacted with another individual in an area with a current measles outbreak.

Members of the unvaccinated general public who have direct contact with an infected individual have a 90 percent chance of becoming infected. The virus can live on a surface for two hours after exposure from an infected host, so even having been in the same location is a potential source of infection. Local health-care providers disseminate a confirmed measles case notification to any health-care facilities or schools that the infected individual attended. A press release may be needed when transmission could have occurred in a public place and locating the exposed individuals is not feasible.

Measles outbreaks at schools and childcare facilities require special consideration. Daily surveillance of all children and staff is needed to assess and reduce the potential spread of measles. Any child or staff member presenting with a fever or rash should be considered contagious and vacate the premises immediately to seek medical attention.

MEASLES IN TODAY'S SOCIETY

The CDC reported over 700 confirmed measles cases from January 2019 to April 2019 in Arizona, California, Colorado, Connecticut, Florida, Georgia, Illinois, Indiana, Iowa, Kentucky, New Hampshire, New Jersey, New York, Oregon, Texas, Tennessee, and Washington. This outbreak is the most significant quantity of cases since 1994. The resurgence of measles in specific communities is probably due to the substantial number of children who are not vaccinated and international travelers who return to the United States after measles exposure.

Today, hot spots of measles outbreaks result from parents not vaccinating their children for philosophical or religious beliefs supported by law. Forty-four states and Washington, DC, provide religious exemptions for school immunizations. Fifteen states offer exemption for personal beliefs, including Oregon, Idaho, Utah, Arizona, Colorado, North Dakota, Oklahoma, Texas, Minnesota, Arizona, Louisiana, Wisconsin, Michigan, Ohio, and Pennsylvania. Idaho has some of the highest rates of confirmed cases, especially in rural areas. Nearly 20 percent of all kindergartners are not vaccinated. Vaccination hesitance is attributed to the prevalence of anti-vaccination campaigns. All states reported isolated outbreaks of measles in 2018–2020.

A 2015 outbreak in Mexico, Canada, and multiple states reported 147 confirmed cases of measles attributed to one unvaccinated tourist. New Zealand also struggled with a recent epidemic and had 639 confirmed cases by August 2019 (Manhire, 2019) with an additional 2,194 cases in 2020 (National Measles and Rubella Laboratory, 2021). A teenager from New Zealand contributed to a multistate outbreak in the United States in August 2019. The contagious teen tourist visited Disneyland, Universal Studios, and other tourist locations in California. The teenager developed the classic measles rash shortly after visiting California and potentially exposed hundreds of people. The public health authorities reported that this scenario could be catastrophic, as measles is the most contagious virus in the world and 90 percent of unvaccinated persons exposed to the virus will contract the disease within one to three weeks. Public health officials tried to locate and notify everyone with whom the teenager had come into physical contact.

Senator Richard Pan, a California pediatrician, wrote and supported state Senate Bill 277, which outlawed anyone working or attending a public school from receiving a vaccine exemption for philosophical or religious beliefs. This law reversed the previous MMR vaccine exemption, which allowed for an exception with documentation stating that receiving the vaccination violated the person's personal view. This bill was passed into law in 2015. California only supports unvaccinated children attending public schools with a medical exemption at this time, such as immune deficiencies that would make getting vaccinated a health risk. However, employees of public schools have not received training to thoroughly vet the medical exemption documents, allowing for potential loopholes. A 2018 outbreak in the San Francisco Bay Area was traced to an unvaccinated teenager who traveled internationally and exposed several children with questionable medical exemptions after returning to the United States.

A large community of unvaccinated Orthodox Jews in New York State, New York City, and New Jersey had a devastating outbreak in 2018–2019. A total of 242 confirmed cases were identified. The person who originated the infection, or *patient zero*, was an unvaccinated adult who had traveled to Israel. Israel was experiencing an outbreak at the time, with 3,150 confirmed measles cases, primarily children. An Israeli doctoral student conducted a research study to determine the reason for not inoculating the children. The informal qualitative research inquiry comprised five mothers of unvaccinated children within the community who had contracted measles. Reasons for not vaccinating their children included cultural and religious principles and the confidence that God was in control of the illness, not a vaccine (Otterman, 2019).

There continues to be a struggle between the medical and ethical issues surrounding vaccination in today's society. The crux of the situation surrounds whether parents should be able to refuse vaccination for their children due to their personal or religious beliefs. Most people opposed to vaccinating their children believe that this is a personal decision and that the government should not force vaccinations on their children. Many unanswered ethical issues surround vaccinations. However, measles was eradicated from the United States in 2000, and with consistent inoculations, this could be achieved again. The question is, should the government and health-care officials mandate vaccinations for all children, regardless of personal beliefs?

2

The History of Measles

The disease of measles, also known as rubeola, has been a part of human history for thousands of years. Initially, smallpox and measles were considered the same illness, but Muhammad ibn Zakariya al-Razi (865–925 CE), or Rhazes, a Persian doctor, discovered characteristics of measles that separated the two infections. His discoveries earned him the title of the father of pediatrics. This highly contagious disease measles stems from the rinderpest virus, which originated from cattle. Immunologically naïve populations have been reduced and—in some cases—eradicated by measles because it is a persistent endemic disease for many geographical areas and among some defined peoples. This disease has had the potential of being destroyed with a practical and consistent worldwide vaccination agenda. Exposure to measles was considered a regular life event for children until relatively recent times, the 1960s. The measles vaccination crusade of 1963 substantially reduced infection rates, and measles was virtually eliminated from the United States by 2000. However, global anti-vaccination campaigns have resulted in a resurgence of this disease.

CATTLE HERDERS IN THE MIDDLE EAST: THE ORIGINS OF MEASLES

Scientists speculate that measles infections date back to the Epipaleolithic period (20,000–10,000 BCE), the middle portion of the Stone Age when people survived as hunter-gatherers. This phase of nomadic activity came to a gradual end as the weather changed to colder and drier conditions. Humankind transitioned to agriculture and domesticating herd animals, such as goats, sheep, and cattle. The domestication of herd animals forced people to live in settled communities with close proximity to enclosed pastures to protect livestock from predators. This practice offered safety for the animals but exposed the human population to animal-specific diseases and viruses.

Animal-specific viral families known as *Paramyxoviridae* produce the morbillivirus and rinderpest virus, both of which infect a broad array of animals. The morbillivirus resides in humans, primates, cats, dogs, bears, weasels, and hyenas, and rinderpest is a primary virus among buffalo and cattle. Scientists have determined that measles diverged from the rinderpest virus, also known as the "measles of cattle," through detailed genetic sequencing and the molecular clock analysis (used to predict the evolutionary timeline for when biomolecules diverged during prehistoric times). Divergence enables a virus to evolve into a new species or subspecies via viral evolution, a combination of biology and virology that renders a rapid mutation. It is the ability of viruses to quickly mutate in response to changes within the host's environment. Scientists postulate that most viral species have common ancestors that evolved into our contemporary infections based on viral evolution.

Measles and smallpox were considered the same disease in ancient eras. Historical writings indicate that a viral disease with a rash and sores caused thousands of people to die in various cultures and countries. This confusion has led historians to believe that while periodic measles outbreaks occurred between 430 and 426 BCE, there is no conclusive evidence that supports the presence of an epidemic. The Bible mentions a "plague," reframing an undescribed illness that caused a multitude of deaths. Archaeologists and scientists have extrapolated smallpox DNA remnants from human remains dating back to the tenth century CE, but measles does not allow for paleopathological evidence in human remains. This makes it impossible to determine the first measles outbreak. The historical evidence suggests that this disease emerged during the Stone Age and affected multiple regions and populations.

EARLY TREATMENTS

Physicians and faith healers of the third century CE failed to distinguish smallpox and measles as different diseases. Both were highly contagious and presented with a rash and sores. In 340 CE, Ko Hung, a Chinese chemist, discovered differences between the two infections, but the treatment for both remained the same. Hung's beliefs were confirmed 300 years later in Egypt by a Christian priest known only as Ahrun (640 CE). Many early physicians and faith healers persisted in treating measles and smallpox as the same disease. Initial treatments included herbal remedies, bloodletting, and exposure of affected areas to heat to burn off the rash and sores. Rudimentary poultices applied to an infected person were heated to draw out the infection.

Progress on measles and smallpox treatments improved through the scientific rigor of the Persian physician Muhammad ibn Zakariya al-Razi (865–925 CE), also known as Rhazes. Rhazes was also a philosopher and alchemist, and he is considered the father of pediatrics. Rhazes wrote over 200 books on medicine, religion, alchemy, and philosophy. Several medical textbooks written by Rhazes profoundly influenced European and Western medical schools for centuries. In his book *Man la Yahduruhuu al-Tabib* (For One without a Doctor), he offered medical guidance for those who did not have access to a physician, including how to identify symptoms and the treatment of various illnesses.

Rhazes's book *Al-Judari wa al-Hasbah* was translated into Latin, Greek, and eventually English as *A Treatise on Smallpox and Measles*. This book provided the first accepted medical explanation of the specific characteristics distinguishing between the two diseases. He offered observations on the disease's progression, specifically the cutaneous (skin) and systemic symptoms. Rhazes rejected the classical Greek physicians' claims that smallpox and measles were the same disease based on his pediatric clinical observations. The book addressed three specific strategies for treating measles: general health, diet, and topical ointments. The patient's overall health plan included sipping cold water and sniffing essential oils, such as sandalwood and camphor. Still, the patient was cautioned to avoid bathing, sexual intercourse, and hot weather. Nutritional recommendations included cold foods (lentils, cabbage, pomegranate, etc.) while avoiding sweet fruits such as figs and grapes. Further, the patient was to gargle with pomegranate juice if a rash developed in the mouth and throat. Rhazes also proposed that massage and sweating helped expel the infection from the body, and washing with cold water was considered essential to reduce the outbreak's pain and duration. The suggested diet especially took into consideration the progress of the signs and symptoms: for example, at the beginning of the incubation period, the patient should address the "hot temperament," or fever, with cold foods and ingest prunes for constipation.

The early treatment of measles was rudimentary and based on access to herbs and foods. This practice is the foundation for Eastern medicine. The World Health Organization (WHO) supports many Eastern medicine practices dating back over 2,000 years. Such traditional methods utilize herbs and plants to cultivate a healthy immune system and treat symptoms. Lentils have proven antioxidant properties, and cabbage is a known probiotic that has proven effective in fighting viral diseases. The herbal practices include using *talbina*, a traditional Iranian food that is high in carbohydrates. Talbina has anxiolytic and antidepressant qualities that improve and stabilize moods. Khodabaklsh et al.'s article "Measles from the Perspective of Rhazes and Traditional Iranian Medicine: A Narrative Review" (2016) mentions that the herb reduces the anxiety of measles's itchy and painful rash.

Today, physicians and scientists are revisiting the efficacy of traditional medicine against measles, such as vitamin A. Vitamin A is now part of the evidence-based practice for measles in the United States. This protocol came about in response to the discovery that vitamin A reduces the symptoms of viral infections. Research is currently assessing the benefits of pyrrolizidine alkaloids used by the Chinese as an antiviral treatment. Japanese research has garnered compelling evidence that anti-fever herbs, such as elderflowers, catnip, yarrow, echinacea, and lemon balm, are useful as antipyretics (medications that lower a person's temperature). Many advances in modern health care are supported by traditional medicine in advancing the prevention and treatment of measles.

CHRISTOPHER COLUMBUS BRINGS MEASLES TO THE AMERICAS

In 1492, King Ferdinand (1452–1516) and Queen Isabella (1451–1504) of Spain sponsored a voyage across the Atlantic Ocean for the Italian explorer Christopher Columbus (1451–1506). Columbus sailed across the Atlantic Ocean in the galleon ships the *Niña*, the *Pinta*, and the *Santa Maria*, seeking a faster route to India. Instead, he connected the Old World of Europe and Africa with the New World of the Americas. The explorer brought religion, wine, seeds for crops, and animals to initiate European settlements in the New World. Unfortunately, he also delivered novel diseases such as typhoid, flu, smallpox, and measles. Pre-Colombian Native American tribes had been living encapsulated within a controlled environment, exposed to few disorders, rendering them defenseless against the illnesses that traveled with Columbus and his seafaring crew members. The uninhibited microbes swept through the tribal populations. Death was so extensive that 80–95 percent of the population died during the first 100 years after the first contact.

Christopher Columbus then traveled to the Caribbean island of Hispaniola in 1492, at which time the island's census was approximately four million inhabitants. The devastation caused by a viral infection within the

Taino and Carib populations caused them to diminish to fewer than 100,000 on the island. By 1570, virtually the entire Taino community (who had been conscripted by the Spanish as slaves to work in the gold mines) on the island was almost extinct. This pattern of depopulation was also seen in Cuba around 1511 when the Spaniards arrived.

Historian Alfred Crosby (1931–2018) coined the term *Columbian Exchange* to depict the Old and the New Worlds' reciprocal relationship, both known and unknown. The European continent benefited from discovering staple crops such as potatoes, maize, and peanuts. Along with these new products, new diseases also entered Old World civilizations and ravaged Europe, Africa, and Asia, with infectious syphilis and tuberculosis being prevalent. Although syphilis is not usually deadly, it produced a change in social discourse throughout Europe. Tuberculosis, on the other hand, had a high mortality rate and was challenging to treat. Many historians believe that the illnesses Christopher Columbus brought back from the New World were deadlier than the Black Death that swept through Europe in the 1300s. The reciprocal relationship between the Old and New Worlds was an amalgam of positive and negative consequences. Still, the most significant was the decimation (both accidental and intentional) of Native Americans.

EPIDEMICS IN THE PACIFIC ISLANDS

The Pacific Islands are in the oceanic region that extends from the Arctic Ocean at its northern border to Asia, Australia, and South America. Sixteen countries are within its boundaries, and it houses over 2,000 islands, some of which are only one square mile. Isolated from foreign visitors, the Pacific Islands slowly became inhabited by Western civilizations as part of the shipping routes. The exposure of measles to these isolated populations as a first-contact viral infection caused high mortality rates across all ages. A major epidemic of measles with its distinctive skin rash ravaged the islands of Hawaii, Fiji, Tonga, Samoa, and Rotuma in the early 1800s. Approximately 25 percent of the entire Pacific population died from measles. The mortality rates were higher on the smaller and distant islands because the adults affected by measles were gravely ill and unable to care for their infected children. The Pacific Islands depopulation continued from 1824 to1848 in large part due to the high mortality rate of measles.

Measles symptoms in the Pacific Islands ranged from acute inflammatory gastritis to severe and lethal hemorrhages due to thrombocytopenia. Thrombocytopenia is a condition that systematically decreases blood platelets and reduces the ability of the person's blood to clot. This condition increases the risk of bruising or bleeding. Interestingly, most measles deaths in the Pacific Islands were from gastrointestinal complications (ileocolitis, diarrhea, and dysentery) instead of respiratory issues, the most common complication for other populations. Measles, unfortunately, continued to jump haphazardly throughout much of the Pacific Islands over the next century. The mortality rate began to decrease when vaccinated travelers visited the islands and the population of islanders with natural immunity increased.

Hawaii

In the 1700s, Hawaii was a series of remote islands rarely visited by foreigners. The English sea captain James Cook (1728–1779) began to explore the islands in 1778. It was not a pleasant visit. The ruler of one of the Hawaiian Islands attempted to steal one of Cook's ships, and in retaliation, Cook tried to kidnap the ruler. During the scuffle that ensued, Cook was killed. After this event, the Hawaiian Islands culture began to change with regular visits from European explorers and Christian missionaries. The visitors brought many new diseases that resulted in the deaths of over 175,000 islanders in short order.

The Hawaiian King Kamehameha I (1738–1819) overtook all the Hawaiian Islands and united them under his governance. The Kamehameha I realm flourished and had a consistent arrangement of visitations by European explorers and missionaries. Kamehameha I died in 1819. He was succeeded by his firstborn son, Kamehameha II. Kamehameha II was intrigued by European culture and wealth. King George IV was equally fascinated with the Hawaiian culture. He gave Kamehameha a ship as a gift, much to the dismay of his family and court members. In 1823, Kamehameha and one of his wives set sail for England in their gifted ship to pay their respects to King George IV. The royal couple arrived in England for an unannounced visit in 1824. Although King George IV was intrigued by Hawaiian culture, he was not receptive to the surprise visit and avoided meeting the royal couple. Historical records indicate that King George IV proclaimed that he would not sit at the table "with such a pair of damned cannibals." The rigid English court concurred with their monarch and considered the Hawaiians to be uneducated and uncivilized.

The English press recorded that the Hawaiian royal couple visited the city's zoo and a local puppet theater. They had become the most talked about couple in England. Kamehameha enjoyed cigars at several public locations. Historians believe that the royal couple contracted measles during a visit to the Royal Military Asylum, the official orphanage for the children of military families and was known to be full of childhood diseases. Because Hawaii and other Pacific Islands were geographically remote and immunologically naïve to many Western diseases, such as measles, the royal couples were defenseless in fighting the virus. Both King Kamehameha and his wife developed the classic red rash, fever, and other measles symptoms and rapidly became deathly ill. The couple died within a month of arriving in England and never met King George IV or any other English royal family member.

Island of Rotuma

The island of Rotuma initiated a strict quarantine because of measles outbreaks on surrounding islands. However, in 1911, a foreign ship was allowed to anchor off the island, and passengers came ashore. Among the passengers were two women who had been diagnosed with measles but did not have the classic red rash. They were allowed to disembark and visit the island. The women would have been contagious four days before presenting a rash and four to five days after the rash disappeared. During this infectious period, the two women exposed almost the entire Rotuma population of 2,616 to measles, and approximately 13 percent of the Rotuma population died. The ship's medical officer kept detailed medical records and provided insight into the events that followed the initial exposure. The immunologically naïve Rotuma populous had a high mortality rate due to its geographic isolation and minimal exposure to outsiders.

Fiji Island

Political upheaval among Fiji's tribal leaders led to articles of secession from the British Empire. This process necessitated that the senior chief, Cakobau, travel with his son and several other chiefs to Sydney, Australia, in 1874. After completing the British Empire's political process, the party returned to Fiji in January 1875 aboard the warship HMS *Dido*. All sixty-nine top-ranking chiefs attended a celebration of secession from Great Britain. A sizable welcoming party boarded the vessel upon its arrival in Fiji and escorted the party ashore. The leaders then returned to their perspective islands to disseminate the legislative changes to their people. They also brought back more than political news; they were contagious with measles and exposed hundreds to measles throughout the Fiji nation when they returned to their respective islands.

The historical records indicate that one of Cakobau's sons became ill during the return voyage, but the origin of the illness was uncertain. Cakobau's son died from measles shortly after the celebratory event. His father became gravely ill and was bedridden. In the Fijian culture, it was customary to pay homage to high-ranking officials, especially a chief, so hundreds of people visited the dying chief in his bedchamber. Everyone who did so was exposed to measles.

The Fijian population suffered a loss of one-fifth to one-fourth of its people by June 1875. Almost all the chiefs died, leaving a political vacuum during a crucial time in their history, when Europeans were expanding their shipping routes in the Pacific Islands.

Samoa

The measles outbreak of 1918 within the small country of Samoa was devastating. Samoa and New Zealand have a unique historical relationship; Samoa was under New Zealand's administration from 1914 to 1962. During this time, the relationship offered public resources and unrestricted travel between the two countries. Most children of Samoa who traveled between the two countries were unvaccinated, and both countries had low vaccination rates. This situation posed a considerable risk for any unvaccinated children when traveling between the two countries. The New Zealand government was aware of a measles outbreak in 1918, but it did not contain the disease's spread or inform the Samoan government. The explosion of infections resulted in a large-scale international effort to inoculate and care for the infected children, but it was too little too late. Hundreds of Samoans died from measles, especially children under five years of age.

GERM THEORY

People of early civilizations believed that foul odors could produce a disease, or "evil spirits." The general population thought that severe illness and premature death were supernatural events caused by a spell or demonic possession. Childhood mortality in the 1700s to 1800s was 43.3 percent, according to Our World in Data (2019). Parents rarely saw all their children enter adulthood due to a lack of understanding about the causes and treatments of viral infections, even well into the modern eras. The life expectancy was only thirty-eight to forty-four years of age.

Superstitions continued to dominate the cultures until the development of germ theory. Athanasius Kircher (1602–1680), a Jesuit priest, is credited with first using the microscope to identify germs, or "worms," found in people who had contracted the plague in the 1600s. He proposed that the microorganisms, or germs, seen with the microscope were the cause of illness. The germs invade humans or animals and begin replication within the host.

The French scientist Louis Pasteur (1822–1895) was influential in the scientific advancement of vaccines with his contributions to germ theory. This theory is currently the most accepted scientific explanation for many diseases. It states that pathogens (germs) are microorganisms that lead to infection. The organisms are too small to see without magnification but can invade humans and develop a host relationship from one species to another. His research with germ theory assisted in the creation of a vaccine that made a significant impact on reducing deaths in humans from rabies. Pasteur conducted experiments in the 1800s with pasteurization that demonstrated how live microorganisms in the air cause food and liquid spoilage. Exposing the food or liquid to mild heat (100 degrees Celsius) eliminates harmful pathogens and extends its shelf life.

Pasteur's discovery supported the germ theory of disease and was further explored by the scientist Robert Koch (1843–1910), whose stance was that live organisms caused disease. Germ theory of disease declares that microorganisms, known as pathogens, can result in disease. Koch conclusively proved that a particular germ resulted in a specific condition by examining anthrax incidence among cattle. Anthrax can be found naturally in the soil and is consumed by cattle. Koch used a microscope to view the blood cells of cows that had died from anthrax and found a rod-shaped bacteria. He then injected this contaminated blood into mice, who subsequently developed anthrax. Animals with anthrax succumb to a quick but agonizing death. The animals experience respiratory and cardiac distress, followed by convulsions and death. Fortunately, the disease progresses very quickly, and most animals are found dead.

Koch's discovery led to the formulation of four postulates that directly link conditions to germs: (1) the bacteria is present with the disease, (2) the microorganism must be cultured from the host, (3) inoculation with the culture must recapitulate the disease, and (4) scientists must then match the organism back to the original microorganism. Postulate three is arguably the most important, as it states that an infection reproduces when inoculated into a healthy host. Modern scientists still accept this theory to explain how viruses mutate from one species to another.

A GLOBAL ENDEMIC DISEASE

Measles has been an endemic disease for hundreds of years as an ongoing and permanent illness for a geographic region or population at a consistent baseline without external influence. The two types of endemic diseases are holoendemic and hyperendemic. A hyperendemic condition has a continuously high contagious rate among all genders and ages. A holoendemic disease affects everyone within a specific geographical area.

Measles is a holoendemic disease in the United States and in many countries.

As a holoendemic disease, measles traveled across isolated geographical areas and devastated populations with no natural immunity from the 1400s to the 1800s. The Danish physician Peter Ludwig Panum (1820–1885) conducted extensive research on the measles epidemic in Iceland and Norway during the mid-1800s. Several years prior, a measles outbreak swept through the two countries, and 75 percent of the populations of Iceland and Norway had exposure to measles; almost all the infected died. Dr. Panum noted that none of the elderly population (over sixty-five) had been infected or exhibited any symptoms during the outbreak. He postulated that the older adults did not contract the infection because of an ability to defend the body against the virus's second exposure. This hypothesis was confirmed in every village that Dr. Panum observed.

Today, over twenty million measles cases occur annually on a global basis. The organization Our World in Data (2019) reports that 45 percent of childhood deaths are from infectious diseases, including measles. Measles is preventable with a low-cost vaccine. The WHO estimated that the measles vaccine prevented over twenty-one million deaths in Africa alone from 2010 to 2017. However, it remains one of the leading causes of death among children.

Most developing countries have managed to mitigate their measles endemic status but have outbreaks in isolated geographical locations. Developing countries continue to battle endemic measles. Some countries are economically unable to provide adequate immunizations or lack the governmental infrastructure to advance an immunization plan. The coronavirus (COVID-19) pandemic has reduced the physical and financial resources of many countries to vaccinate for measles and COVID-19 simultaneously.

1963 MEASLES VACCINE

Vaccines have a long history of fighting human infectious disease, dating back to 1000 CE when the Chinese developed a smallpox inoculation using live smallpox material but with little success. The first effective smallpox vaccine was a homegrown recipe by a cattle breeder in England named Benjamin Jesty (1737–1816). In 1774, a smallpox epidemic hit his rural village. Jesty had already recovered from having smallpox, which he believed was because of his consistent exposure to cows with cowpox. He therefore decided to inoculate his wife and children with material from a cow that had cowpox. His entire family survived the smallpox epidemic and showed no signs of any side effects from smallpox. Jesty was not interested in making his discovery known, and only a few people were aware of what he had accomplished. His wife was very proud of his development and had his tombstone inscribed with "the first person who introduced the cowpox inoculation." This historical event spawned considerable interest in live viral inoculations and gained the attention of an English physician named Edward Jenner (1749–1823).

Edward Jenner (1749–1823), known as the pioneer of immunizations, was determined to develop vaccines to eradicate smallpox and measles. He continued to explore a smallpox vaccine by building on previous research, such as using genetic material from an infected cow in 1796. Jenner injected fluid from a smallpox blister and applied it to the skin of an eight-year-old boy named James Phipps. The child developed a blister for a short period but no other symptoms. Jenner then inoculated the boy with smallpox matter, and he had no response from the injection. Thus, the vaccine was a success. The success of the smallpox vaccine was the impetus for creating additional immunizations, especially for measles. Jenner described the pathophysiological effect vaccine in his 1798 report titled "Inquiry into Causes and Effects of the *Variolae Vaccinae*, or Cow-Pox."

Jenner's successful smallpox vaccination prepared the groundwork for French physicians Charles Nicolle and Ernest Conseil, who discovered that patients exposed to measles developed antibodies against the disease. They hypothesized that this could offer people immunity against subsequent measles exposure in the 1900s. Dr. Peebles, a World War II bomber pilot who became a physician, presented compelling evidence for this theory in 1954. Dr. Peebles collaborated with his colleague, Dr. John F. Enders, on researching a measles outbreak among school-aged children in Boston, Massachusetts. The gentlemen collected blood samples from all the ill children to isolate the measles virus. It is documented that the physicians told each boy, "Young man, you are standing on the frontiers of science. We are trying to grow this virus for the first time. If we do, your name will go into our scientific report of the discovery."

The scientists ultimately succeeded in this endeavor within a month with the blood of a thirteen-year-old boy named David Edmonston. The scientists dubbed the blood sampled as their "Edmonston B strain" of measles virus and began the process of developing a live-attenuated (weakened) strain of the virus from the blood. The scientists needed the vaccine to cause the immune system to be initiated and create antibodies that would fight the measles but be weak enough to produce minimal to no side effects. Inoculations began in 1958 at Fernald School and Willowbrook State School for disabled children. The vaccine proved too potent, so most children developed a rash and fever, similar to measles. Some of the children had extremely high fevers that caused seizures. The vaccine was termed toxic, and subsequent research sought to invent a vaccine that would be safe to administer. The investigation led scientists to a method of growing the microorganisms in eggs, and a second vaccine was simultaneously given with measles antibodies to lessen the side effects.

John Enders and his fellow scientists achieved the goal of producing a safe and effective attenuated measles vaccine in 1963. Distribution began in 1968 with the Edmonston-Enders measles vaccine, and it has remained the only vaccine used in the United States. The vaccine is usually a combination vaccine that protects against measles, mumps, and rubella (MMR) or measles, mumps, rubella, and varicella (MMRV).

Public health officials and physicians administered a different version of measles vaccine for a short period between 1963 and 1967. This version did not have the live-attenuated measles virus but a "killed" virus. The killed version did not provide equivalent protection and was subsequently discontinued. The Centers for Disease Control and Prevention (CDC) recommends that those who received this version of the vaccine or are unsure of the type of immunization they received must have an additional vaccination. According to the CDC, everyone should receive at least one dose of the live MMR for maximum protection, and minimal risk is involved in receiving further treatment with the MMR shot. Until the measles vaccine was created, nearly everyone contracted measles, and "people accepted a measles diagnosis as a part of life," according to Dr. Graham Mooney (2011), an associate professor at the Institute of the History of Medicine at the Johns Hopkins University.

2000 U.S. ERADICATION CAMPAIGN

Measles became a notifiable disease in the United States in 1912; all health-care providers and facilities were required to report all confirmed and suspected cases to public health authorities. The first decade of reporting was shocking! Over 6,000 measles-related deaths occurred each year, totaling 60,000 lives lost in the United States by a preventable disease. The CDC set a goal to eradicate measles from the United States. This goal was not achieved, but the disease rate was reduced by 80 percent from the previous year.

Eight years later, this positive trend did not continue; numerous outbreaks among school-aged children prompted the Advisory Committee on Immunization Practices, the American Academy of Pediatrics, and the American Academy of Family Physicians to formally recommend a second dose of the MMR vaccine for additional protection. Reported measles cases continued to decline following this recommendation, and the disease was declared eradicated in 2000.

Eradication was due to the highly effective vaccination program and stricter controls implemented on international travelers coming to the United States. The implemented travel controls originated from the WHO, who stated that it would be safe for travelers to enter any geographical regions that had documentation showing no endemic measles within that geographic area for one year. The region must have had a surveillance system with a successful track record of identifying measles cases. This policy does not mean that measles has wholly disappeared or that a child or adult will never have measles in the United States. There are still travelers who continue to bring measles into the country and expose unvaccinated children and adults in isolated areas. The United States' eradication status would be eliminated if an outbreak continued for more than one year. According to the CDC, it is expected that isolated episodes will continue to occur in the United States. Still, most of the population is protected because most of the population is vaccinated, a clear example of the herd immunity discussed in chapter 1.

ANTI-VACCINATION MOVEMENT

The anti-vaccination movement has a long history of conflicting beliefs between those who support vaccination and those who are opposed. Historians report the first immunization (known as variolation) occurred during the Chinese Song dynasty (960–1279) for smallpox. The live smallpox virus injected into the skin produced milder symptoms than the naturally occurring disease. The smallpox mortality rate improved from approximately 2 percent to 30 percent during this period.

Dr. Angelo Gattis (1730–1798) introduced the smallpox vaccine in France in 1763 but did not achieve promising results, as there were severe side effects and high mortality rates. The French Parliament outlawed inoculations shortly after the practice began. In 1796, successful treatment in England for smallpox was still considered a controversial practice. Most English people did not trust the modernization of medicine or those who called themselves a doctor. The clergy reinforced this fear, proclaiming smallpox as God's punishment, and said it should not be prevented or treated.

Additional failed attempts to produce vaccines against cowpox and smallpox spurred mistrust of all vaccinations. In England and the United States, anti-vaccination leagues formed that resisted the immunization of children in the late 1800s. The institutions waged several court battles to repeal any mandatory vaccination laws but had little success. Public health officials in Cambridge, Massachusetts, enacted a law in 1902 that required all residents of the city to vaccinate against smallpox. Most of the city's population complied with the law, but one man refused and appealed in court. The courts determined that each state could enact and regulate rules on compulsory immunizations. The U.S. Supreme Court upheld the lower court's decision based on each state's need to protect its citizens from infectious diseases.

In England, the Vaccination Act of 1853 formalized the anti-vaccination controversy. Immediate resistance resulted in the formation of several organizations, the most prominent being the Anti-Vaccination League. One member of this league was William Tebb, who traveled to the United States in 1879 to proclaim vaccines' detrimental effects. Due to Tebb's influence, anti-vaccination associations in California, Wisconsin, and Illinois initiated court battles to repeal compulsory vaccination in those states. Despite the success of many vaccines against polio, typhoid, influenza, and whooping cough, many were still wary of vaccine safety. This fear was reinforced in 1955 when 120,000 cases of the Salk polio vaccine were found to contain a live virus, resulting in over 40,000 confirmed polio cases, 53 cases of paralysis, and 5 deaths.

Additional safety issues continued with the diphtheria, tetanus, and pertussis (whooping cough) vaccine. This vaccine was associated with thirty-six children suffering from neurological conditions at London's Great Ormond Street Hospital. Sweden reacted to this incident by issuing a pertussis vaccine moratorium for seventeen years, during which time over 60 percent of Swedish children contracted pertussis before the age of ten.

The anti-vaccination movement rapidly escalated in the 1900s. Mobs formed at health-care facilities to prevent public health nurses from inoculating children. Vaccinations for polio and smallpox began to decline due to the public questioning the safety of the medications. Additional distrust grew when the Salk polio vaccine was mistakenly manufactured with a live poliovirus, resulting in over 40,000 cases, with 53 children developing permanent paralysis and 5 dying. The most devastating blow to vaccination rates happened in 1998 when a British doctor published a research study linking the MMR vaccine with bowel disease and autism. The research was later deemed fraudulent in 2011 and retracted by the publisher (*The Lancet*) that had printed the original article; even so, public opinion on the MMR vaccine had been permanently tainted. Media outlets continue to spread unsubstantiated material related to vaccinations. Chapter 9 will describe additional issues with the MMR vaccine and provide an in-depth exploration of the anti-vaccination movements in today's society.

3

Causes and Risk Factors

This chapter will explore the cause of measles and its contagious properties. Measles is contracted through exposure to a contagious person or through direct physical contact with airborne particulates or contaminated surfaces. Physical or face-to-face exposure provides the optimal scenario for the spread of the virus. The infected person coughs or sneezes into another's face, and the infected respiratory droplets are inhaled. Once inhaled, the virus travels into the person's nose and throat, where it begins replication. The cough or sneeze contains tiny aerosolized particles that can stay suspended in the air for long periods after the person has left a room, and the virus can live on surfaces for up to two hours. What worries health officials is that measles virus can be spread four days before the onset of the telltale rash, so people with the virus start being contagious before they have any symptoms or even know they have measles. Scientists have determined measles is not viable on soft surfaces or spread through clothing. The transmission must be from direct exposure of aerosolized droplets, physical contact, or touching a hardened surface that harbors the droplets.

Infected persons are often unaware that they are exposing others to the illness because they have no symptoms that would cause them to suspect that they are ill. The contagious period is as much as four days before the rash associated with measles is evident. Other symptoms with measles, such as coryza (runny nose) and cough, are often associated with other illnesses, such as allergies and the common cold, which increases the risk of spreading the disease during the prodromal period.

THE CAUSE OF MEASLES

Measles is an infectious illness caused by the rubeola virus. As a single-stranded RNA virus, it is a member of the *Morbillivirus* genus in the *Paramyxoviridae* family. Viral replication occurs in the throat or nose of the host, and it is disseminated through respiratory droplets. The tiny droplets contain millions of contaminated particles that can easily be spread to the general public. The virus requires a host, and humans are the only natural host for measles. The illness is spread through physical contact, airborne particulates, or contaminated surfaces. The following paragraphs will detail how measles is transmitted.

PHYSICAL CONTACT

Measles is a highly infectious disease that will affect 90 percent of non-immune people who have direct contact with a contagious person. It is an aerosolized virus, meaning it invades an infected person's saliva and respiratory secretions. The contaminated secretions are released into the air when a person talks, sneezes, or coughs. People become infected after they have had direct contact with the mucus or saliva of a contagious individual. The virus can then enter the body via the eyes, nose, or mouth and contaminate the respiratory tract. Close physical contact (within twenty-four inches) and conversing with an infected person allows the aerosolized droplets to be projected into the eyes, nose, or mouth. Even being exposed to the breath of a contagious individual provides the opportunity for viral droplets to enter a person's body.

AIRBORNE EXPOSURE

Airborne exposure allows the virus to spread uninhibited from person to person. Even with casual face-to-face contact, a person can become infected with measles because there is no control over who has breathed in that airspace. A person with measles can talk, sneeze, or cough in a room, and aerosolized droplet nuclei containing the virus are suspended in the air; secretions that contain live viral contaminants have been cultured for up to two hours after the infectious person had left the room.

The risk of exposure (and consequences) for unvaccinated people increases in closed areas or areas with poor ventilation, such as a waiting room in a dentist's or doctor's office. Being on an airplane, bus, or automobile with closed windows further increases the risk of contamination due to restricted air circulation. The virus can be suspended in the air for up to two hours after the expulsion, and the actual amount needed to become infected is relatively small. All it takes for viral replication to take place is for a core of measles single-stranded RNA to fuse with a host cell membrane, penetrate the cell body, and begin replication. Viral replication typically starts in the respiratory tract's epithelium cells, starting with the nasopharynx (nose and mouth).

Another entry route for the aerosolized droplets is the eyes. The eyes' conjunctiva is a suitable site for a viral invasion via the myeloid or lymphoid cells. The conjunctiva is the outer membrane of the inner eyelid and eyeball. The viral exposure initiates an inflammatory response, causing the small blood vessels to dilate and become more visible, hence the pink or reddish appearance of the eye(s) commonly known as pink eye. Symptoms include pain, redness, tearing of the eyes, and itching. Conjunctivitis generally responds well to antibiotic ointments or eye drops if treatment begins in the early stages.

A sneeze can travel farther than most people think! Researchers at the University of Bristol in England found that the average sneeze travels through the air at 100 miles per hour and contains an average of 100,000 contagious germs. These germs are most contagious during the initial expulsion and the next one to three minutes. The expelled droplets' size contributes to the potential risk of invasion of the respiratory tract, specifically the lungs. The smaller the droplet, the deeper it can travel within the body, according to Allen Haddrell, a PhD researcher at the University of Bristol. Most respiratory pathogens, including measles, measure less than a human hair (120–150 nanometers in diameter) and have the potential of traveling some distance due to air movement. Air movement, including central air-conditioning or wall units, facilitate the particles in traveling longer distances and increase additional exposure.

CONTAMINATED SURFACES

The virus can also survive on hard surfaces for up to two hours. The virus resides in the contagious person's respiratory tract—specifically the throat and mouth. When the contagious individual coughs or sneezes, contaminated droplets travel through the air in an arched trajectory and land on hard surfaces. The uninfected person risks exposure by coming into contact with the dirty surface and then touching their nose, eyes, or mouth.

Hard surfaces, defined as impervious surfaces, allow the aerosolized matter to remain on the material's outer layer and not be absorbed. Soft surfaces have not been found to transmit measles because the viral particles are absorbed into the material. On the other hand, sometimes the respiratory droplets are visualized as fine sprinkles of liquid. The internal environments of homes, schools, and health-care facilities are filled with hard surfaces such as tables, desks, and chairs. Even toys made from plastics meet the definition of a hard surface. An aqueous (water-based) solution containing germicidal bleach is required to clean hard surfaces. The Environmental Protection Agency (EPA) recommends one cup of bleach to four cups of water to disinfect hard surfaces and the use a soft cloth to wipe down the total exposed area. Then allow the surface to air-dry. Other practical options include disinfecting wipes for home use and germicidal wipes for health-care facilities.

AT-RISK POPULATIONS

At-risk populations are individuals who, due to their age, gender, frailty, race, economic status, or health history, are at an increased risk of infection or disease. For measles, the at-risk population includes infants, unvaccinated children, unvaccinated adults, pregnant women, immunocompromised children, anyone with poor nutrition, and those with a vitamin A deficiency. The unvaccinated population under the age of five and over the age of sixty-five is exceptionally vulnerable.

Infants

Infants (less than one year of age) automatically receive natural protection against measles from the mother during pregnancy, but this protection decreases over the infants' first year of life. This natural protection is why the Centers for Disease Control and Prevention (CDC) and the World Health Organization (WHO) recommend that the first dose of MMR vaccine be administered at one year, when the naturally acquired antibodies have disappeared and the infant is now susceptible to the virus. Some people mistakenly believe that the current vaccination schedule could place an infant's life in danger; that is not true. The recommendation is based on the time frame that the vaccine would benefit the infant the most.

Children

Unvaccinated children under the age of five have an increased risk of getting measles, especially when traveling outside their local community in the United States or internationally. The CDC reported over 1,000 measles cases in thirty-one states in 2019. This figure represents the highest number of cases since measles was declared eradicated. Most of the confirmed cases were in New York State and in geographical pockets of unvaccinated children with religious waivers. However, the risk increases exponentially with international travel to areas currently having a measles outbreak. Obviously, areas with a current outbreak will increase the opportunity for measles exposure through physical contact, airborne exposure, and contaminated surfaces.

Measles is more common in the winter and spring, when sniffles and sneezing are rampant. Children often have poor hygiene habits and touch or hug others after coughing or sneezing. They usually do not cover their mouths when coughing or sneezing, increasing the risk of airborne exposure and contaminated surfaces. Both hygiene habits can increase the risk of spreading the virus as it lands on surfaces in the classroom. According to the CDC, a single unvaccinated child who sneezes or coughs within a closed classroom can expose twelve to eighteen other children. This exposure rate is exponentially higher than most other viruses, including the human immunodeficiency virus (HIV), severe acute respiratory syndromes (SARS), and even Ebola. One Ebola case usually results in two infected people, while HIV or SARS often leads to four additional positive cases. Kindergartens and elementary schools that historically accept unvaccinated students have often experienced a localized outbreak with devastating results.

Unvaccinated Adults over the Age of Sixty-Five

Mature adults over the age of sixty-five are at higher risk for several complications from measles. Measles symptoms will begin with the typical feeling of fatigue and cold symptoms. The hallmark facial rash begins within five days, spreading to the torso, arms, and legs. The symptoms can rapidly progress to life-threatening difficulties, such as pneumonia (lung infection) and encephalitis (brain swelling). The National Foundation for Infectious Diseases reports that mature adults tend to have an increased risk of severe complications due to comorbidities or other health-care concerns that reduce their immune response or increase infection risk. One predominant peril is the thirty-four million Americans diagnosed with diabetes, as reported by the Diabetes Research Institute. Diabetes increases the risk of infection and prolongs recovery. Other chronic conditions afflicting the elderly, such as hypertension (high blood pressure) and cardiovascular disease, intensify measles's adverse effects.

Pregnant Women

Most women of childbearing age are vaccinated against measles, mumps, and rubella, and therefore their infants are protected against these diseases. Although measles does not cause congenital disabilities, the virus does increase the risk of medical complications requiring hospitalization, including pneumonia. Testing for rubella is routinely performed for women considering becoming pregnant. A positive result confirms immunity. A negative test result indicates that measles vaccination is needed.

Unvaccinated pregnant women are advised not to receive the MMR vaccine until after delivery; this waiting period is because the MMR vaccine contains live-attenuated (weakened) viruses. This procedure contrasts with most other vaccines because they use a killed virus. Doctors usually advise avoiding pregnancy for at least one month after receiving the vaccine due to the vaccine's attenuated viral load to reduce the risk of becoming infected. Exposure to a nonimmune pregnant woman may cause health problems for both the mother and her unborn baby. According to a CDC study, the mother's most common associated effect was pneumonia, and the most common fetal or neonatal outcome was premature delivery or low birth weight. If the exposure is within the ten days before delivery, this will likely cause a severe infection in her newborn at birth.

Immunocompromised People

People with compromised immune systems, including those with HIV, cancer, or poor nutrition, are considered at high risk to contract measles. Both HIV and measles cause immunodeficiency within the host. HIV leads to progressive immunodeficiency at the cellular and humoral levels. T lymphocytes initiate an attack within the cell membrane. Humoral immunodeficiency utilizes antibodies from the B cells to bind with antigens, destroying or breaking the invading cells through lysis. Humoral immunity occurs in body fluids. Measles only uses cellular-mediated immunity and does not result in a progression of the immunity-related illness. Measles presents with flu-like symptoms that are similar to HIV.

Leukemia Patients

The CDC reports that people with weakened immune systems from leukemia are incredibly vulnerable to all vaccine-preventable diseases, including measles. This risk does not exclude those who are vaccinated. The treatment for leukemia is chemotherapy. Chemotherapy reduces the response of the immune system. One study conducted in New Zealand by the Ministry of Health in 2012 suggests that the abnormal decline continues for three years. So, even children that received their two-dose vaccination can contract measles. Physicians recommend that children and adults be reimmunized following their chemotherapy program.

Those with Poor Nutrition and Vitamin A Deficiency

Poor nutrition increases the risk of adults and children contracting measles and post-measles syndromes, according to Dr. P. Bhaskaram (1995). Dr. Bhaskaram has researched the correlations between nutrition and measles since the 1990s. He reports that poor nutrition accounts for 3–4 percent of secondary infections and deaths associated with measles.

The CDC reports that poor nutrition and vitamin A deficiency leads to severe measles-related complications, extended recovery time, and ocular (eye) damage. Severe complications include encephalopathy (brain swelling) and pneumonia. While most children recover from measles in ten to fourteen days, this vulnerable population may have symptoms that linger for months or result in permanent damage. The permanent damage is often xerophthalmia, a corneal ulcer, or permanent blindness. Xerophthalmia is dryness on the eye and lack of tears, which causes conjunctivitis. A vitamin A supplement is the primary treatment, either by injection or pill. Another complication is corneal ulcers, which are sores on the front of the eyes that appear as white dots. While they usually respond well to topical ointments, opaque scar tissue may be a long-term injury that can inhibit vision or cause blindness. Another potential complication is nutritional keratomalacia, resulting in blindness. Antibiotic therapy and vitamin A offer protection from these concerns; however, these remedies are often unavailable to those with socioeconomic restrictions.

4

Signs and Symptoms

The symptoms of measles are relatively consistent for every person and are defined as the three C's, which include coughing, coryza (runny nose), and conjunctivitis (inflamed eyes), in addition to fever and rash. The three C's are specific signs that measles has entered the respiratory tract. The incubation period of measles is specific to each person, generally seven to ten days after exposure. Of course, this is based on the length of exposure and the viral load of the contagious individual. Other symptoms associated with measles include gastrointestinal and neurological deficits.

INCUBATION PERIOD

The World Health Organization (WHO) defines the incubation period for measles as between ten and fourteen days, but it can be seven to twenty-three days from exposure to symptom onset. The prodromal (initial) phase begins with malaise and a high fever, followed by a cough, conjunctivitis, and coryza. The hallmark maculopapular rash presents two to four days after the initial symptoms or ten to twelve days after exposure. The rash may appear as early as seven days from exposure and as long as twenty-one days from exposure. Many factors affect the incubation period, including the overall health status and age of the exposed individual.

A person is considered contagious for approximately four days once the rash has appeared and will continue to be contagious for four to five additional days after the rash disappears. Due to the benign nature of prodromal symptoms, many people do not recognize that they may have been exposed to measles because these symptoms are generic to many other illnesses. It is not until the appearance of the telltale rash that measles is considered a diagnosis. The exposure source is often unknown, as an infected person can be in the prodromal stage while being contagious to others. The symptoms are vague during this stage and difficult to link to a positive measles diagnosis; however, the infected person can spread the illness to 90 percent of unimmunized individuals. Due to this rampant exposure rate and variable incubation period, measles is considered one of the most contagious diseases. A person can spread it without any knowledge that they have been infected.

THE THREE C'S

Three common symptoms, known as the three C's, cough, coryza, and conjunctivitis, are consistently associated with measles. However, the symptoms are generic enough to indicate that the body is "fighting something" as the immune system begins its assault on the virus. All three could result from a common cold or the beginning of various respiratory infections, but with measles, they predict a potentially severe illness.

Cough

Tussis, or a cough, is a voluntary or involuntary reflex the body uses to expel fluids, mucus, microbes, irritants, and foreign particles from the respiratory tract. The act of coughing is a rapid and forceful air expulsion from the lungs, up the trachea (windpipe), through the pharynx, and out through the mouth. The cough reflex is an attempt by the body to clear the respiratory pathways of obstruction. Several irritants may initiate a cough reflex; for example, smoking is a prevalent cause resulting in a distinctive chronic cough, especially in the morning. Measles is associated with a dry, hacking cough that begins around the seventh day of measles exposure. The cough is often described as an annoying tickle sensation.

An article titled "The Present and Future of Cough Counting Tools," by Hall et al. (2020), was presented at the third International Cough Conference; it advises physicians to use the cough counting method to classify a cough. This methodology provides an excellent way to evaluate the severity of a person's cough. The Hull Automatic Cough Counter (HACC) analyzes the digital recordings of coughs using a cough counter. This enables physicians and pulmonologists to appropriately dispense antitussive medications, especially for the pediatric population. Phone applications are available to the general public for a nominal charge. Although a relatively new option for physicians, the HACC is becoming increasingly popular for distance health care, such as telehealth.

Coryza

Coryza, also known as rhinitis, is inflammation within a person's nasal mucous membranes. There are numerous causes for a runny nose, including a cold, allergies, and respiratory infections. The most common symptoms are congestion, watery discharge from the nares (nostrils), sneezing, and postnasal drip. There are several effective natural remedies for a runny nose suitable to both children and adults. The most effective treatment of coryza is drinking plenty of fluids, mainly water, which can prevent dehydration and reduce overall feelings of congestion. The fluids thin out the congestion and make it easier to expel. Failure to consume adequate fluids causes thick and tenacious nasal discharge. It is best to avoid liquids such as coffee and alcoholic beverages, as they can lead to dehydration.

Conjunctivitis

Conjunctivitis results from an infection or inflammation of the conjunctiva. This transparent membrane lines the eyelid and the sclera (the white portion of the eyeball). When the conjunctiva becomes inflamed, small blood vessels become more visible and give the eye a reddish or pink appearance. This discoloration is why conjunctivitis is commonly known as pink eye. Conjunctivitis is extremely contagious through contact with eye secretions. Conjunctivitis is a hallmark sign of measles when a person also exhibits a fever, cough, and runny nose. This symptom often occurs before a rash appears and abates when the virus has run its course.

GENERAL SYMPTOMS AFTER EXPOSURE

Measles can cause a number of other signs and symptoms, many of which are considered complications of the disease (see chapter 6 for more information). These include the well-known measles rash.

Fever

The medical terminology for fever is pyrexia; any temperature above 100.4 degrees Fahrenheit is considered a fever. This temporary condition can be the result of myriad internal and external anomalies. The thermostat for the body is in the hypothalamus of the brain. The hypothalamus shifts the temperature from the normal range (97–99 degrees Fahrenheit) to signal the immune system. With measles, the fever indicates a viral invasion. The fever appears seven to fourteen days after the initial exposure and lasts from four to seven days.

Children with even a slight fever (99–100.5 degrees Fahrenheit) are symptomatic, which can indicate a severe illness. Most physicians support the belief that fevers are beneficial in combating diseases and do not treat the fever with medications. Fevers signal the immune system to initiate disease-fighting cells to begin attacking infections. Others recommend using over-the-counter antipyretics, such as acetaminophen, ibuprofen, or naproxen. Fevers can often be reduced with cool baths and cold packs in the groin area and under the armpits. This practice should only be used temporarily for children and adults who can communicate any discomfort.

A fever is expected with measles but is not necessarily a reason to seek medical treatment. Parents need to contact their pediatrician when an infant younger than three months has a fever resistant to cool baths and antipyretics and is over 100.4 degrees Fahrenheit. Infants between three and six months with a rectal temperature greater than 102 degrees Fahrenheit and who exhibit pain or lethargy need to be evaluated by a doctor. Infants older than six months with a fever and any additional symptoms may need to be seen by a doctor based on their symptomology. Children with a fever who can still drink and play do not need to be seen by a doctor, but if they become irritable, complain of a headache or stomachache, or have a fever that lasts longer than three days, medical attention should be sought.

Adults can tolerate fevers without too much discomfort unless the fever is more significant than 103 degrees Fahrenheit. Adults with a fever greater than 103 degrees should try cold baths and over-the-counter medication first and seek immediate medical treatment if changes in mental or neurological status, vomiting, seizures, stiff neck, or abdominal pain present. Adults with measles should anticipate having a fever and diligently monitor for symptoms. Adults often have spikes in their temperature that indicate severe symptoms requiring hospitalization.

Respiratory Symptoms

Otitis media is the most common respiratory complication resulting from measles. The ear is connected to the eustachian tube via the upper respiratory tract, providing a direct pathway for viruses to reach the lungs. Fourteen percent of children under five years of age in the United States will present with an ear infection (otitis media) as a side effect of measles. The epithelial cells within the eustachian tube obstruct a response to measles exposure. This obstruction results in a secondary bacterial infection. Children over the age of five and adults have reduced rates of otitis media due to the larger diameter of the eustachian tube.

Croup, or laryngotracheobronchitis, with measles was present in 9–32 percent of hospitalized children in the United States, according to the Centers for Disease Control and Prevention (CDC). Most of the affected children had bacterial pathogens cultured from their trachea and presented purulent exudate. Laryngotracheobronchitis is the second most common cause of death for children over the age of five, and pneumonia is the most common measles-associated death for hospitalized children. The reason can be a direct result of measles or a secondary viral or bacterial infection associated with the measles virus. Studies indicate that approximately 50 percent of children had mild radiographic changes, and 77 percent had moderate to severe changes. Progressive pneumonia is the most common cause of death for immunocompromised persons of any age with measles.

Gastrointestinal Symptoms

A loss of appetite in a child is often a symptom that parents identify first. The loss of appetite and lack of fluid intake increases the likelihood of dehydration, which is further complicated with diarrhea, affecting one out of ten people with measles. Scientists suggest that diarrhea associated with measles is a twofold occurrence. The virus targets the epithelial cells that line the body's cavities and organs and reduces the immune system's effectiveness. Stool samples of children with measles-associated diarrhea have the same bacteria as stools from children with diarrhea not linked to measles. The results suggest that the initial onset of diarrhea is related to a suppressed immune system, which appears in conjunction with the appearance of a rash. The secondary bacterial infection is due to immunosuppression and changes to the epithelial surfaces as the culprit of long-term and severe diarrhea.

Prolonged diarrhea has been the most common complication among fatal cases of measles in underdeveloped countries. Several studies have found a definitive link between prolonged diarrhea and increased mortality. Children who present with prolonged diarrhea often have difficulty achieving the typical growth pattern of their peers. Dehydration is a potentially life-threatening problem that can directly result from severe diarrhea but is most often due to several factors. According to the World

Health Organization (WHO), people with malnutrition, vitamin A deficiency, and immunosuppression are at higher risk for measles-associated diarrhea, dehydration, and mortality.

Neurological Symptoms

Febrile seizures occur in 1–3 percent of children diagnosed with measles. These seizures are usually benign and episodic. Febrile seizures are a convulsion caused by a spike in temperature, usually from an infection. A temperature higher than 100.4 degrees Fahrenheit can produce seizures (jerking) of the arms and legs with a loss of consciousness. A simple febrile seizure lasting fewer than fifteen minutes is the most common. A complex febrile seizure lasts longer than fifteen minutes, and several episodes can occur within twenty-four hours. Parents are advised to call 911 and seek emergency treatment with any seizure.

Maculopapular Rash

A maculopapular rash is composed of flat and raised skin lesions. These individual lesions eventually merge together, creating one large rash. This rash usually appears three to five days after the onset of symptoms and lasts about a week. Individuals usually feel most ill on the first or second day after the rash's appearance.

Although the maculopapular rash is probably the best-known and most distinctive symptom of measles, it is important to note that this type of rash can occur as the result of other bacterial or viral infections, an allergic reaction, or medications.

Koplik's Spots

Peculiar small white spots—called *Koplik's spots*—with a reddened background may appear on the buccal mucosa (the inner cheek area inside the mouth) near the first and second upper molars. The sites may occur two to three days after exposure without any other symptoms. The appearance of Koplik's spots is a pretty clear indication of exposure to measles. Physicians and public health officials use this diagnostic approach to identify measles and initiate isolation of contacts with early surveillance. Both actions aid in the control of measles during the prodromal period.

Dr. Henry Koplik (1858–1927), an American pediatrician, is credited with this discovery. Dr. Koplik began his medical practice as a pediatrician in Berlin, Prague, and Vienna before he returned to New York City and worked with poor European and Jewish immigrants in the Lower East Side. The early nineteenth century was ravaged by various contagious and deadly illnesses, one of which was measles. The treatment of infectious diseases was complex during this time, and diagnosing them was even more troublesome, but Dr. Koplik rose to the challenges of studying measles symptoms. It was common knowledge that a patient with the classic maculopapular rash had measles and was contagious before the rash appeared. What Dr. Koplik was searching for was a definitive symptom that occurred before the rash. He found the clue in 1896 by following detailed histories and physical examinations. Three days before the appearance of the rash, odd bluish-white spots had appeared in the buccal (cheek) area in every patient's mouth. This oddity brought international fame for the physician and served as a method to combat future epidemics.

Koplik's spots were used to provide the doctor with a quick diagnosis when his son came down with measles. One of Dr. Koplik's sons developed a cough, runny nose, and fever, but no rash, while traveling on an ocean voyage to Europe with his mother and siblings The ship's physician examined the child's mouth, discovered the bluish-white spots inside the cheek, and diagnosed the boy with measles. The most exciting part of the story is that the ship's physician recognized the signs because he had read a medical journal by Dr. Koplik, the child's father. According to the physician's records, the child recovered from measles without any residual complications.

5

Diagnosis, Treatment, and Management

The diagnosis, treatment, and management of measles are directly related to the patient's presentation. The health-care provider will assess the symptoms exhibited and decide whether the person has measles. Symptoms include the three C's, cough, coryza (runny nose), and conjunctivitis (inflamed eyes), with a fever and rash. If needed, a titer, or blood test, is performed, but this is rarely used in the United States. The treatment for measles-associated symptoms aims to reduce discomfort with prescribed medications, over-the-counter medications, and home remedies. The management of measles employs measles genotyping to track the transmission pathway during outbreaks. Genotyping mitigates the number of those infected and the duration of the epidemic. Of course, the most effective management tool is the isolation of the contagious person.

DIAGNOSIS

A diagnosis of measles is based on a clinical case definition of the disease, which consists of standard medical criteria for the classification of specific diseases and syndromes used in international surveillance of the disease. It is essential to epidemiologists that a standard is established and maintained to quantify and report all measles cases. All clinical case definitions have three essential variables: person, place, and time The *person* designates key characteristics that patients have in common—for example, age, occupation, sex, or race. The *place* describes a specific geographical location (city or community) or facilities, such as nursing homes or hospitals. *Time* delineates a period associated with the onset of the illness. By limiting the time, similar conditions are excluded and not considered in the surveillance.

The World Health Organization's (WHO) clinical case definition is any person of any age who has a fever, maculopapular rash, cough, coryza, and conjunctivitis. The person must have all these symptoms simultaneously to be clinically confirmed as having measles, with or without laboratory confirmation. If the physician doubts the diagnosis, a laboratory confirmation called a *titer* can be performed. A positive measles titer is considered epidemiological proof, but the WHO does not require laboratory confirmation for a legitimate measles diagnosis; it may be based on the presence of clear qualifying indicators such as signs and symptoms.

The Centers for Disease Control and Prevention (CDC) has identified measles as a nationally notifiable disease. All confirmed or suspected cases must be reported to the appropriate public health departments. The *Manual for the Surveillance of Vaccine-Preventable Diseases* (2014) provides health-care providers and public health practitioners with policies and guidelines in this matter. The case definition for measles found in chapter 7 of the CDC's surveillance handbook offers a general clinical description of a person with an acute illness characterized by a temperature greater than 101 degrees Fahrenheit with a cough, coryza, and conjunctivitis. The person will exhibit a maculopapular rash approximately three days after the symptoms begin. Anyone with these symptoms should be isolated and considered to be a "probable measles case." Probable cases are evaluated by an epidemiological link or confirmation with laboratory testing. The CDC definition states that anyone with an acute febrile (fever) presentation, a rash, and a positive serologic (blood) test for measles antibodies (IgM) is a confirmed case. A person with a positive titer does not need to have a fever or a rash. Confirmed cases are questionable if an MMR vaccination had been received in the previous forty-eight days because of the live virus used in the injection.

Laboratory Testing for Measles

Laboratory testing for the rubeola virus is conducted with a serologic test, a throat or nasopharyngeal swab, and a urine specimen. According to the CDC's *Manual for the Surveillance of Vaccine-Preventable Diseases* (2014), both forms of specimens detect measles-specific IgM antibodies and measles RNA. Serum samples should be collected during the acute phase or at least three days after a rash appears. In a few cases, samples taken before the appearance of the rash may have a false-negative result because the antibody response is too weak to be detected, for which a second serum sample is recommended. The desired volume of blood is 0.5 to 1 milliliter; this amount allows for retesting. The minimal amount of blood is 0.1 milliliter of blood for one test. The blood must not be frozen but stored on ice at a consistent temperature and centrifuged within two hours after collection to separate the serum. The blood is transported in sterile tubes with a threaded cap and sealed with an O-ring. The blood should be immediately stored on ice and shipped to the appropriate public health facility. Blood from infants and children may be obtained by a finger or heel stick.

Throat and nasopharyngeal swabs are successful in detecting measles when collected on the first day of the rash and up to three days after the appearance of the rash. A flocked polyester fiber swab is the commercial product recommended for collecting samples. Cotton swabs are not recommended because they often contain a substance that inhibits laboratory analysis. Once the sample has been collected, the swab is placed in a standard viral transport medium consisting of a sterile isotonic solution and a protein, usually 0.5 percent gelatin, which is required to optimize the content of the sample. Samples without a protein stabilizer will reduce the infectivity by 90–99 percent, thereby rendering the specimen nonviable. The wood or plastic portion of the swab can be broken or cut to allow the swab to be completely contained in the storage container. Samples must be maintained at 24.8 degrees Fahrenheit and shipped within twenty-four hours.

Urine samples can be used to confirm a measles case but are generally the last choice. A volume of fifty milliliters of urine must be collected in a sterile container. The urine is then centrifuged for fifteen minutes and stored with cold packs. The CDC recommends freezing the urine for transport and shipping in a sealed container with dry ice.

Genotyping

Measles virus genotyping is the process used to track transmission pathways during outbreaks. Genotyping links the virus among confirmed cases of wild-type viruses. Wild-type measles is a naturally occurring viral infection with eight clades (A to H), indicating that the viruses have a single common ancestor. The measles virus's ancestor is the rinderpest virus, which was derived in the eleventh and twelfth centuries from cattle. The WHO's Measles and Rubella Laboratory Network (LabNet) performs standardized testing in over 183 countries to identify genetic characteristics.

This global database has functioned for more than twenty decades and placed over twenty-three recognized genotypes. The agency was initiated in response to a worldwide resurgence of measles. The mission of the organization revolves around the development of quality control programs for virologic surveillance activities.

Scientists distinguish between naturally occurring measles and reactions to the live-attenuated vaccination through the process of genotyping to identify the source of measles, which is essential during outbreaks. The viral strain can be traced to a particular country, geographic area, and often to *patient zero*, the person who initiated the outbreak. Once genotyping has been used to obtain this information, surveillance and notification processes begin, preferably early in the episode, so that health officials can reduce the number of potential victims and reduce complications. Confirmed measles cases must be genotyped in countries that have virtually eliminated measles. A reference stock of all known measles strains is held at two separate gene banks. The Division of Viral Diseases (DVD) of the CDC (cdc.gov/ncird/dvd.html) in Atlanta, Georgia, and the Virus Reference Department (VRD) of Public Health England (PHE) in London, England (https://www.gov.uk/government/collections/virus-reference-department -vrd), are overseen by the WHO.

TREATMENT OF THE THREE C'S ASSOCIATED WITH MEASLES

There is no known cure for measles because it is a viral infection that does not respond to antibiotics or antivirals. The only treatment is specific to the symptoms exhibited by the patient. Antibiotics will not have any effect on measles. However, they are routinely ordered for secondary bacterial infections. Antiviral medications are helpful for some viral infections, but this does not include measles. To date, no antiviral has been approved by the Food and Drug Administration (FDA) to combat measles.

Cough

The act of coughing is a rapid and forceful expulsion of air from the lungs, up the trachea (windpipe), through the pharynx, and out the mouth. The cough most associated with measles is an annoying dry cough, but it may become so severe that it causes the person to lose his or her breath or results in chest pain. The nonproductive, or hacking, cough is an involuntary reflex to expel fluids and irritants from the respiratory tract. There are numerous nonpharmaceutical treatments for the cough associated with measles; the most common is drinking hot tea with honey. Hot liquids open up the airway passages, as does inhaling the steam, and honey is a well-known natural remedy that soothes the irritated membranes of the throat.

One pediatric study by Paul et al. (2007) published in *Pediatric Adolescent Medicine* compared the effectiveness of honey to the over-the-counter cough suppressant dextromethorphan as a double-blinded study during which parents completed a survey for two consecutive nights. All participants began the first night with no interventions, but on the second night, each of the 105 child participants received one of three treatments: honey, honey-flavored dextromethorphan, or no treatment. Significant improvement was reported by parents who administered a single dose of honey thirty minutes before bedtime. There was no significant difference noted in children who received dextromethorphan or no treatment.

Over-the-counter cough suppressants in the form of a liquid or lozenges assist in reducing the cough reflex. Cough suppressants are primarily recommended for administration at nighttime to help the person get an extended period of uninterrupted rest by reducing the cough reflex. Over-the-counter cough suppressants such as dextromethorphan reduce the cough reflex in the brain and relieve the cough for a short time.

Other nonpharmacological treatments include using a humidifier to moisten the air and reduce the cough reflex. The same benefits are achieved by taking a hot shower and breathing in the steam. Adolescents and adults can try breathing the mist from a pot of hot water with essential oils, such as eucalyptus. Many people report relief using this method, as it opens up the respiratory passages. However, extreme caution should be used. The steam can cause thermal burns of the face, and supervision is required for all children and adolescents using hot water. Simply drinking hot beverages will temporarily reduce the cough reflex and alleviate throat pain.

Other effective methods of gaining temporary relief include sucking on hard candy and sipping water or juices, as the consumption of water or other fluids is the most common and practical means of treatment. The Mayo Clinic has recommended that the average adult consume two to four liters of fluids every day, primarily water, to maintain homeostasis. Homeostasis is the body's tendency to maintain a constant internal environment. For example, the body tries to regulate body temperature and water levels. When the body is in homeostasis, it is considered healthy and balanced. Water consumption is especially important when ill because the body needs an additional one to two liters.

Evaluations and treatments of coughing have changed over the past few years because verbal descriptions of a cough are ineffective and obscure. Most pediatricians use the Hull Automatic Cough Counter (HACC) as a method of appraising a child's cough. Hull's digital recordings analyze the severity of the cough using a cough counter. The tool can be downloaded onto a smartphone for a nominal fee ($10 to $25), and parents can record the coughing of a child for a prescribed amount of time. The recording and the analysis are then available to the pediatrician for prescribing antitussive (cough) medication. The HACC is a scientifically based option widely accepted for remote health care, such as telehealth.

Coryza

A runny nose, also known as *coryza* or *rhinitis*, demonstrates inflammation in the nasal passages' mucus membranes. The patient experiences a feeling of fullness or congestion in the nose and face. Pain in the face increases if the person bends over. A consistent and uncomfortable watery discharge out the nose is present, which can thicken and change to a white or yellow color if a secondary infection is present. Several nonpharmacological treatments are effective for children and adults suffering from rhinitis. The most effective coryza treatment is drinking plenty of fluids, mainly water, which reduces the overall feeling of congestion and increases hydration. With adequate hydration, fluids thin out the congestion and make it easier to expel. Failure to consume adequate fluids causes a thick and tenacious nasal discharge. It is best to avoid liquids such as coffee and alcoholic beverages, as they can lead to dehydration. Elevating the head of the bed while sleeping can assist in draining fluids from the nasal passages that irritate the throat and produce a cough.

Consuming hot beverages assists in opening up the nasal passages and soothing discomfort from congestion. Some herbal teas, such as chamomile, ginger, and mint, are mild decongestants and have anti-inflammatory properties. Steam from the beverage temporarily helps open up the nasal passages and decreases the effort needed to breathe. Nasal discomfort and cough relief have similar treatments. A hot shower will expand the nasal passages and relieve the person's congestion by expelling the mucus. It is wise to supervise children taking a hot shower; the water temperature can change rapidly and scald the skin. Another treatment that mitigates a runny nose is a facial steam bath; it relieves congestion and thins the mucus. The thinner the mucus, the easier it is for the person to expel it by blowing his or her nose.

A simple and natural method of relieving coryza is with a nasal lavage, often called a *neti pot*. Most pharmacies, health stores, and retail stores offer these tools for a reasonable cost. The pot resembles a small teapot, and it is filled with warm saline water that can be purchased premade or concocted at home by boiling one cup of water with a half teaspoon of table salt for fifteen minutes with a lid on the pot. Once the solution has cooled to room temperature, it is poured into the neti pot to use as a sinus rinse. The saline water is poured into one nostril, and it flows out the other nostril. Only sterile water is used to reduce the risk of a nasal infection. The sensation of a nasal rinse is uncomfortable for many people and can generate extreme coughing. This treatment should be used with caution, especially for younger children.

The chemical capsaicin, which is found in spicy foods, dilates the nasal passages and reduces the pain caused by congested membranes. Several studies have concluded that capsaicin has beneficial effects on relieving nasal symptoms without any significant side effects. If a person cannot tolerate spicy foods, a small amount of ground-up hot peppers mixed with water can be applied to the nose's external areas for the same effects. It is advised that the mixture be tested for a possible reaction before applying capsaicin to the nose.

Pharmacological treatment for a runny nose includes the use of over-the-counter antihistamines. These medications, such as chlorpheniramine and diphenhydramine, block the release of histamines and reduce the symptoms. However, they can cause drowsiness and dry out the membranes of the eyes, nose, and mouth. This sensation is uncomfortable for many and may cause rebound symptoms. Rebound symptoms exacerbate nasal discharge and increase the risk of a secondary bacterial infection. Severe reactions have occurred with antihistamines, including dizziness, visual disturbances, lack of mental clarity, and hallucinations. Stringent monitoring is needed for children and adults when taking an initial dose of an antihistamine. It is recommended to contact the person's primary care physician immediately or call 911 with any severe reaction.

Conjunctivitis

Conjunctivitis, also known as pink eye, results from infection and inflammation on the sclera, which is a transparent membrane lining the eyelid and the white portion of the eyeball. When the conjunctiva becomes inflamed, small blood vessels become more visible and give the eye a reddish or pink appearance, hence "pink eye." Occasionally, a doctor may perform a laboratory analysis (culture) on the eye's discharge if a bacterial infection or foreign substance is suspected. Conjunctivitis resulting from measles ranges from mild to extreme discomfort, so the treatment is based on the severity of the symptoms.

Conjunctivitis is highly contagious and can quickly be spread from one person to another through contact with eye secretions. For example, children with conjunctivitis rub their eyes because of the itching sensation or to remove secretions. Then, they spread the infection through direct contact with another child or by transferring the secretions to a hard surface that another child touches.

A compress, cold or warm, often temporarily relieves the pain. Nonprescription pain relievers are also effective with mild symptoms, and over-the-counter eye drops containing an antihistamine may reduce inflammation. If the symptoms worsen or the physician suspects a person has a secondary bacterial or fungal infection, steroids combined with antibiotic eye drops may be considered. Oral medications to control systemic inflammation, such as a decongestant, are also an option. Artificial tears can alleviate some symptoms, but other over-the-counter eye drops are generally not recommended.

Eye drops are prescribed to alleviate the discomfort of conjunctivitis. The installation of these eye drops requires extreme care, as touching the tip of the dropper on the surface of the infected eyeball will contaminate the solution. The head should be tilted back slightly as the eye looks toward the ceiling. The lower eyelid should be gently pulled down with clean hands to create a pocket for the placement of the solution. The tip of the dropper is held over the eyelid pocket, and the fluid is gently squeezed out to the appropriate number of drops. The eye should be closed with the pad of a finger placed on the inside corner of the eyelid near the nose, pressing gently for a few moments. Any fluids around the eyes can be patted dry with a tissue.

TREATING OTHER SYMPTOMS OF MEASLES

Although having a cough, coryza, and conjunctivitis are the most common symptoms of measles, there are other signs and symptoms associated with this viral infection. This section describes these symptoms and their associated treatments.

Keratitis

Keratitis is the most common secondary infection. It is termed *viral keratitis* when measles causes it. Viral keratitis affects the cornea. The cornea is the clear dome-shaped window located in the front of the eye that covers the pupil (the opening in the center of the eye), the colored part of the eye (the iris), and the anterior chamber (the fluid-filled interior portion of the eye). The cornea functions as a filter for the light entering the eye; it is also a barrier to prevent germs from entering the eye's inner portions. Keratitis requires prompt medical attention to prevent vision loss.

Treatment for viral keratitis is an antiviral eye drop and an oral antiviral medication. However, a corneal scar may result if treatment is delayed or the patient is noncompliant with the medicines. This scar will permanently affect vision and could cause blindness. Removal of a corneal scar requires surgery to restore normal vision.

Koplik's Spots

Moving from the eyes to the mouth, a person with measles will have Koplik's spots. Koplik's spots are considered a diagnostic indicator of measles. Before a skin rash manifests, these peculiar spots are seen in the buccal mucosa (cheeks) inside the mouth and appear as red rings surrounding blue-white lesions. The spots generally fade in less than a week after appearing. Dr. Henry Koplik discovered the spots in the early nineteenth century. He was searching for a definitive way to diagnose measles during the prodromal period—before the rash appears. When a physician sees Koplik's spots in a person's mouth, the person is diagnosed with measles, even if other symptoms are minimal or have not yet manifested.

Treatment of the spots is focused on relieving the symptoms of mild pain in the mouth and throat. The consumption of a soft diet and an increase of fluid intake is generally recommended, unless the afflicted areas are severe or spread to the throat, in which case gargling with a saltwater solution is recommended. An oral anesthetic and analgesic spray containing phenol (e.g., Chloraseptic) provides quick relief by numbing the throat's oral membranes and the back of the throat when symptoms are severe. The painful areas should be sprayed every two to three hours. The solution should be softly swished in the mouth and spit out. The spray should only be used for a maximum of two days; using this solution for longer than recommended can result in contact dermatitis (skin rash), hives, and painful irritation of the mouth. A rare side effect is a blood disorder called *methemoglobinemia*, indicating that the cells carrying oxygen, the hemoglobin, are unable to release the oxygen appropriately. Low oxygen levels can result in headaches, shortness of breath, poor muscle coordination, seizures, and cardiac arrhythmias.

Maculopapular Rash

There is no specific treatment for the rash associated with measles. Most pediatricians and general practitioners recommend bed rest and generic remedies for the symptoms. Generic remedies include getting plenty of rest, an increase of fluids, and isolation for at least four days after the rash has disappeared. The fever can be reduced by taking acetaminophen or ibuprofen,

Calamine lotion is beneficial to soothe the itching associated with the measles rash. The active ingredients are zinc oxide and iron oxide. Zinc oxide is a gentle astringent and bactericidal that has been used for centuries to reduce mild skin conditions that result in an itching sensation. Iron oxide gives the lotion a pink color and is considered an antipruritic, or anti-itch, drug. The combination of both ingredients aids in drying the oozing or weeping from the rash and temporarily relieves pain.

Calamine lotion is safe for children over the age of two and pregnant women. Before the lotion is applied, the skin should be washed with a bar of antibacterial soap, rinsed well, and patted dry. A thin layer of the lotion should be applied to all affected areas and left to dry completely before dressing; the cream can stain clothing. The lotion can remain on the skin overnight except in the case of sensitive skin. Side effects with sensitive skin are a stinging sensation, angioedema (swelling of the skin and superficial tissues), and hives.

ISOLATION

Isolation is considered a treatment for measles, as it creates a barrier between noninfected people and germs. According to the CDC, there are two tiers of precautions to prevent transmission of infectious agents: standard precautions and transmission-based precautions. *Standard precautions* create a barrier when close to the person or handling body fluids, blood, or open wounds. According to the CDC, standard precautions include washing hands, disposing of sharps (blades and needles), respiratory hygiene (cough etiquette), and personal protective equipment (PPE). PPE may include wearing a mask or goggles, gloves, a gown, and shoe covers: PPE provides a physical barrier between infected and noninfected people. It is vital that PPE be donned (put on) and doffed (removed) appropriately to minimize contamination from the contagions. Hand hygiene is performed as the first step of the PPE process. Then, a gown that covers the torso from the neck to knees is worn with ties in the back. An N95 or surgical mask is secured over the mouth and nose based on the manufacturer's instructions. Goggles or a face shield may be worn and adjusted for an appropriate fit. Snug-fitting gloves cover the wrist section of the gown.

Doffing the PPE is the most important step of preventing transmission of an infection, based on instructions from the CDC. The PPE is considered contaminated after use, so the person wearing the articles must follow the exact steps for removing them. The gloves must be removed before exiting the patient's room by grasping the palm of one hand and peeling off the glove, which is held in the still gloved hand. A finger is slid under the soiled glove to pull it off and then both gloves are discarded in an approved waste container. Hand hygiene is performed after untying the gown, and it is removed by only touching the clean inside area of the gown, rolling the gown into a ball, and discarding it. The goggles or face shield may be removed after exiting the room. Goggles should be disinfected for the next use; the face shield should be discarded. The mask or respirator is removed by the elastics or ties and discarded or reused according to the policies of the facility. Hand hygiene is performed again.

Transmission-based precautions are additional steps that must be followed for specific pathogens. There are three categories: droplet precautions, contact precautions, and airborne precautions. *Droplet precautions* are used to prevent contamination from secretions or mucus from the respiratory tract of an infected person. The germs are expelled as droplets into the air when a person coughs, sneezes, or even talks. The germs can travel in these droplets about three feet from the person in an arc-like pattern. Illnesses that meet this criterion include influenza, pertussis (whooping cough), and coronavirus infection. Everyone must wear a mask when exposed to anyone suspected of having these infections.

Contact precautions are those taken to prevent the spreading of germs through touch, including the practice of wearing a gown and gloves. Such practices are required for most cases but are not necessarily all the protection needed for a person with Clostridium difficile or norovirus, which require additional PPE for adequate protection.

Airborne precautions are needed when pathogens are so minute that they can travel or remain suspended in the air for long distances, as would be needed for a person taking care of someone with an active case of measles. Other pathogens that require airborne precautions are coronaviruses, chickenpox, and tuberculosis. These minute germs' ability to travel is so great that hospitalized patients with these illnesses must be sequestered in specialized rooms that prevent the air from entering the hospital ventilation system. These rooms are called *negative pressure rooms*, as the atmosphere is vented out of the hospital through a separate air duct system. When anyone enters a negative pressure room, they must wear a well-fitted respiratory mask in addition to other PPE protocols.

Isolation and quarantine are both used to reduce exposure to others with a contagious disease; the difference is the degree of separation. According to the CDC, isolation is the separation of a sick or contagious person from others within the home- or health-care facility. For example, placing a person who is hospitalized in a private room is a form of isolation, whereas being quarantined not only separates the person from others but also restricts his or her movements to reduce exposure to a contagious disease. Quarantine restriction within a home means that the ill person has his or her own bedroom and bathroom not used by anyone else. All clothing, dishes, eating utensils, and personal items touched by the contagious person must be separated from others in the home. Infants, children, the elderly, and immunocompromised family members should stay at least six feet away from the patient. It would be prudent to wear a mask and gloves whenever exposed to an area in the home inhabited by a person with measles due to the risk of exposure to a contaminated surface. Exposed surfaces should be cleaned regularly with disinfecting wipes or a water-based solution with bleach. One cup of bleach to four cups of water is recommended by the Environmental Protection Agency (EPA) to effectively kill the virus, and all surfaces must be allowed to air-dry before using.

Isolation in a health-care facility is more stringent, especially for measles. Hospitalized patients with active measles must be placed under airborne precaution protocols for a minimum of four days after the onset of the rash, as measles is transmitted via respiratory droplets. A particulate respirator must be worn by everyone entering the room, which is either an N95 respirator or a powered air-purifying respirator (PAPR). The N95 respirators are intended for use in the health-care setting as class II devices regulated by the FDA and CDC. The respirators contain a coating that reduces or kills microorganisms and filters out 95 percent of air particulates.

The N95 respirators fit very close to the face and are designed to form a seal around the nose and mouth. Most health-care facilities restrict facial hair on employees because the hair can hinder the effectiveness of the seal. The size of each N95 mask is checked each year to ensure an optimal fit. The PAPR removes droplets and particles from the air by using a blower to push the contaminated air through a high-efficiency particulate air (HEPA) filter. The HEPA filter is a mechanical air filter that forces air through a fine mesh to capture harmful particulates, including airborne pathogens. Clean air is vented back into the facepiece. While the PAPR is not a true positive-pressure device, it does have some advantages in that it does not require a fit test; most people can readily wear this device. The most common objection to it is feeling claustrophobic. Another advantage is the ability to reuse the PAPR by cleaning it with disinfectant. The hospital-grade N95 is only recommended for single use, but this practice has been questioned with the recent issues with accessing PPE on a large scale due to the COVID-19 pandemic.

6

Long-Term Prognosis and Potential Complications

Complications can occur with measles acquired either naturally or from the measles, mumps, and rubella (MMR) vaccine. Most complications are expected to be mild or minimally uncomfortable. Severe complications are rare but may occur with the first dose of the MMR vaccine and with naturally occurring measles. The immune system is a fantastic system that protects the body from pathogens that could cause illness and infections. The last section of this chapter defines *immunity* and describes the immune system's response when a person acquires wild-type measles or after receiving the MMR vaccine.

COMMON COMPLICATION FOR THE MMR VACCINE

A common complication of the MMR vaccine is a localized reaction at the injection site known as *urticaria*. Urticaria (hives) is triggered by a response to specific allergens that releases histamine and other chemicals into the skin. With the release of histamine, fluid collects under the skin, causing wheals (swollen areas). The raised skin will be pale red and have a pins and needles sensation. Severe itching is often associated with this reaction. Physicians recommend applying hydrocortisone cream to the site to reduce the itching feeling.

A localized reaction at the injection site is normal and does not indicate an allergic reaction to the MMR vaccine. Pain associated with the MMR vaccine injection is responsive to cold packs applied to the injection site for twenty minutes for the first twenty-four hours. A warm bath may help if the pain is uncontrolled after twenty-four hours. Acetaminophen or ibuprofen, in liquid or pill form, is also an option. Children less than six months of age should not be given ibuprofen. Pain is expected at the injection site for several days.

Antihistamines are an effective treatment that works by blocking the effects of histamines and the itchy sensations from a localized reaction of the vaccine. However, a secondary bacterial infection may need antibiotics, especially for children. Children are prone to scratch until they break the skin. Once this occurs, bacteria from the fingernails is introduced, and the area will become infected. Various antihistamines are available and safe for all ages as an over-the-counter medication, but it is advisable to read the label carefully, as with all remedies. Many antihistamines cause drowsiness, which is a safety issue while driving or operating machinery. Other localized reactions to the injection may appear within twenty-four hours. The individual may experience pain, redness, and tenderness at the injection site. The symptoms are a normal response to the shot and are generally mild and transient, rarely lasting longer than three days. The swelling of the lymph glands in the neck or mouth results from the immune system's response to the attenuated virus. The swollen glands may be tender and cause minor issues with swallowing or bending the neck. A physician should evaluate any symptoms that create more than a minor inconvenience.

Fever is a systemic reaction to the MMR vaccine, and approximately 15 percent of recipients will have a slight fever about seven days after the injection. Acetaminophen or ibuprofen is appropriate for children older than six months and adults with a fever of any origin. Anyone with a fever should get plenty of rest, increase fluid intake, and avoid excessive blankets or clothing. A physician should be seen if the fever lasts more than three days, causes extreme lethargy, or is unresponsive to antipyretics (medications that reduce or prevent fever). Antipyretics signal the hypothalamus to reduce the body's temperature, thus lowering the fever.

Carefully monitor a child's temperature. Any fever greater than 103 degrees Fahrenheit can precipitate febrile seizures. The CDC acknowledges a small but known risk that children might experience a febrile (fever-related) seizure in the twelve days after having been given the MMR vaccine. The episodes are transient and short term. No studies have found it associated with the development of future unprovoked seizures or epilepsy. The treatment goal is to control the fever with over-the-counter medications. There is rarely a need to prescribe anti-seizure medications for febrile seizures.

Fewer than 5 percent of individuals who have been vaccinated will have a rash that appears seven to ten days after vaccination and remains for a few days. This itchy rash will be scattered over the body. Cool baths, over-the-counter pain relievers, and hydrocortisone cream can help to relieve these symptoms. Children will be irritable and have a decreased appetite, but these symptoms are typical and resolve in forty-eight hours.

Teenagers and adults receiving their first dose of the MMR vaccine may experience the same symptoms described above with the addition of joint stiffness. The stiffness and decreased range of motion are linked to the rubella portion of the vaccine. The condition is transient for most but may result in temporary arthritis. Postpubertal teenagers and women are more susceptible than men. Stiffness will begin seven to twenty-one days after vaccination and slowly resolves. No residual effects have been reported.

COMMON COMPLICATION OF NATURALLY OCCURRING MEASLES

For naturally occurring measles, a common complication is a middle-ear infection, or *otitis media.* One out of ten children with measles comes down with a middle-ear infection. Middle-ear infections mean that the area surrounding the eardrum has become inflamed and painful. Fluid trapped in the middle ear may result in hearing impairment and a feeling of fullness. Measles often spreads to the ears through the pharynx as the infection enters the respiratory system, during a measles attack this tube allows fluid to collect in the ear and become infected. Severe infections can affect balance and increase the risk of falls and further injuries. Most otitis media cases are based on the severity of the condition, the medical history of the patient, and treatment preferences. Over-the-counter pain medications are usually the first course of treatment. Antibiotics may be a part of the treatment plan if indicated by the physician. Severe infections that go untreated may cause permanent hearing loss.

Gastrointestinal Disorders

Gastrointestinal disorders such as nausea, vomiting, and diarrhea often accompany measles. Diarrhea is the most common complication. The question is, how does an airborne infection cause symptoms within the gastrointestinal tract? The answer is that measles can infect multiple organs because it targets the epithelial (lining of organs), reticuloendothelial (specialized cells that remove dead or abnormal particles), and white blood cells, all of which are widespread throughout the entire body. All three physical components are vital to the immune system for its defense against illnesses.

Children may get watery diarrhea, known as measles-associated diarrhea, because the virus disrupts the epithelial surfaces of the gastrointestinal tract. This usually occurs just before the appearance of the maculopapular rash; however, stool cultures taken from children with diarrhea not associated with measles show the same bacterial content as cultures taken from children with measles. Leading experts believe that immunosuppression is a secondary culprit that opens the door to a bacterial infection. Other gastrointestinal disorders are related to the destruction of the epithelial surfaces combined with immunosuppression. The disorders include pancreatitis, hepatitis, and stomatitis. The potential for these conditions to become serious depends on the individual's nutritional status and overall health.

Respiratory System Disorders

As an airborne virus, measles will directly affect the respiratory system. Measles can lead to inflammation of the larynx (voice box) and the passageways of the lungs, resulting in laryngitis. Laryngitis causes the voice to become hoarse, and the sufferer has difficulty talking. Voice quality may change from mild hoarseness to total loss of the voice. Treatment is primarily self-care, such as voice rest, increased fluid intake, and breathing in humid air. Inflammation in the bronchial (lungs) tubes may lead to bronchitis and increased difficulty breathing. The person will have a productive and persistent cough due to the mucus in the lungs. The edema (swelling of the respiratory tract) may be so severe that wheezing occurs. Symptoms may continue for weeks until the bronchial tubes heal.

Infants and young children may get an upper respiratory infection that obstructs breathing and causes a cough that sounds like barking. The condition is called *croup*, and it happens when the larynx becomes inflamed and the trachea (windpipe) swells. Croup often resolves with home care, but it is a miserable time for children. They will have trouble swallowing, resulting in a decreased appetite. Their distress can be relieved by placing them in a warm, moist bathroom to relax the airways. A humidifier with a cool mist can also reduce the swelling.

Pneumonia with Measles

Pneumonia is the most common complication of measles. Pneumonia is an infection of the lungs that causes the lungs' alveoli (air sacs) to fill up with fluids or pus. The alveoli are the structures that facilitate the exchange of oxygen and carbon dioxide. Oxygen is moved from the lungs to the bloodstream; simultaneously, carbon dioxide is removed from the blood and exhaled. The exchange happens in the lungs by the alveoli and small blood vessels called *capillaries*. It is challenging to facilitate the oxygen and carbon dioxide exchange or to breathe effectively when the alveoli are full of liquid or pus. The person will have a productive cough, chest pain with breathing, fatigue, loss of appetite, and shortness of breath. If pneumonia becomes severe, a decline in mental awareness occurs. Pneumonia from a virus will not respond to antibiotics. Respiratory support (oxygen), fluids, and rest are prescribed. Recovery is often a long-term process and may take months. Immunocompromised people are especially susceptible to pneumonia, and it may be fatal to this population.

SERIOUS COMPLICATIONS FROM THE MMR VACCINE

Several rare adverse events have occurred after receiving the MMR vaccine; a person may have a life-threatening hypersensitivity response known as anaphylaxis. Anaphylaxis activates the immune system to release chemicals that dilate (enlarge) blood vessels and cause fluids to leak into the surrounding tissues resulting in a rapid drop in blood pressure and edema. Spasms in the larynx (throat) and respiratory tract cause difficulty breathing. The response to this is sudden and dramatic. Anaphylaxis occurs in fewer than ten million MMR doses, but the person's symptoms can lead to death without immediate treatment. Until recently, anaphylactic reactions were suspected to derive from severe egg allergies. Eggs are used as the medium to grow the virus for the MMR vaccine. Case reports show that most anaphylaxis reactions are associated with the gelatin used as a stabilizer in the vaccine. An egg allergy is no longer considered a contraindication.

Idiopathic Thrombocytopenic Purpura (ITP)

Studies have confirmed a causal relationship between idiopathic (or immune) thrombocytopenic purpura (ITP) and the MMR vaccine. The risk of developing ITP within six weeks after receiving the MMR vaccine is 1 in 21,000 based on a study published in the British *Journal of Clinical*

Pharmacology (Blach, Kaye & Jick, 2003). ITP is a blood disorder characterized by a decrease in platelets. Platelets are the cells made in the bone marrow that stop bleeding by forming a clot. The bone marrow is responsible for making all the blood cells, including platelets. Bone marrow continues to produce platelets in all conditions, but blood tests reveal decreased blood platelets in ITP. An average platelet count ranges between 150,000 and 450,000, but with ITP, the number of platelets is fewer than 100,000. The risk of uncontrolled bleeding is substantial in this range. It appears that the immune system no longer recognizes platelets but does recognize the blood cells as an antibody against the attenuated measles virus in the MMR vaccine.

The exact mechanism of acquiring ITP has not been established, but the disorder's results are clear. A reduction in this blood cell results in spontaneous bleeding and bruising; severe cases may lead to internal bleeding. The condition will appear suddenly and may spontaneously resolve in several months; however, ITP may last for several years or a lifetime. Women are two to three times more likely to have this disease than men. ITP is not contagious, and each child with ITP will experience different symptoms, which may include nose bleeds, petechiae, purpura, and blood in the mouth and gums. Petechiae are tiny red spots on the skin from capillary bleeding. They cluster together and appear rash-like. Purpura is also blood from the capillaries, but a more significant amount of blood pools under the skin. These areas have reddish-purple colorations that do not blanch when pressure is applied.

Petechiae and purpura are usually not painful but represent abnormal bleeding from a decreased platelet count. ITP will require medical intervention, which usually starts with a steroid to increase the platelet count. Drugs that support the immune system are sufficient for most children, such as gamma globulin. Medications that stimulate the bone marrow to make additional platelets are usually ordered. A life-threatening consequence of ITP is severe bleeding into the digestive tract or brain. Most children go into remission and remain symptom-free with treatment.

Atypical Measles Syndrome

Immunocompromised adolescents and adults may develop atypical measles syndrome (AMS). This syndrome was first reported after 1,836,000 immunizations with a killed vaccine were given in the United States between 1963 and 1967. A few of these immunized children were diagnosed with this syndrome. The symptoms include fever, rash, and pneumonia; however, there are subtle differences. A study conducted by Dr. E. Mark Nichols (1979) for the CDC in California resulted in developing case criteria that included an atypical rash. This rash was a combination of petechiae and vesicular and urticarial components. Petechiae are small red spots in the skin from bleeding. A vesicular rash has a red tapioca-like appearance with painful blisters. The urticarial rash, or hives, is an itchy raised rash. The rash begins on the extremities as opposed to the hairline and face, as would be the case for regular measles. Koplik's spots are not present with AMS. Most scientists concur that AMS is a hypersensitivity response to measles.

Guillain-Barré Syndrome

Several cases of Guillain-Barré syndrome (GBS) have followed receipt of the MMR vaccine. This rare neurological disorder causes the immune system to attack the peripheral nervous system. Symptoms of GBS include abnormal feelings that begin in the feet and travel bilaterally up the legs. Overall weakness is the major complaint as the disease progresses. Profound weakness will occur by the third week, followed by difficulty breathing and neurological pain (pins and needles) that increase at night. The symptoms may become so severe that the person is paralyzed and needs a mechanical ventilator to breathe. Although some experts support a causal relationship between the MMR vaccine and GBS, the U.S. Institute of Medicine has rejected this correlation. The institute supports the belief that GBS is an autoimmune disorder for which the MMR vaccine does not initiate.

Transverse Myelitis and Acute Disseminated Encephalomyelitis

In 2014, the Food and Drug Administration (FDA) added two additional adverse reactions to the MMR vaccine's label: transverse myelitis and acute disseminated encephalomyelitis (ADEM). Transverse myelitis is inflammation along the spinal cord that damages the insulating material that covers the nerve cell fibers known as the myelin sheath. This function is crucial to the well-being of the body, as the spinal cord transmits messages from the body to the brain for interpretation: For example, when a person touches a hot stove, the nerves of the hand send a message to the spinal cord, which forward the information to the brain. The brain interprets the data and relays a message to move the hand from the stove. Transverse myelitis interrupts this communication process with possibly dire consequences. The person is no longer able to process messages to the brain or receive messages from the brain.

The term *transverse* refers to the band-like sensations in the body's abdomen and chest area. The sensation mimics the feeling of a tight belt or girdle in the abdomen or chest area. Early symptoms include a sharp, shooting pain that wraps around the torso and radiates down the legs and arms. Most sufferers experience weakness in the legs, which can advance to paraparesis (partial paralysis) or paraplegia (complete paralysis) and require the use of a wheelchair permanently. Patients with this condition have paresthesia (abnormal sensations) throughout the body in addition to bowel and bladder dysfunction. Many affected by this condition report generalized flu-like symptoms. All such symptoms can result in diminished overall mental well-being and lead to anxiety and depression. Treatment is symptom based; the goal is to reduce spinal cord inflammation and alleviate the symptoms. Rehabilitation is focused on strength and functionality by reteaching the activities of daily living in ways that promote self-care. Some people recover within a few months; others may take years. Some suffer permanent disabilities that restrict their ability to lead an everyday life.

ADEM resulting from the MMR vaccine is an immune-mediated neurological disorder that causes inflammation of the central nervous system (brain and spinal cord), specifically the myelin sheath that insulates the nerve fibers. ADEM symptoms are sudden and mimic encephalitis symptoms, including headache, stiff neck, fatigue, nausea, and vomiting. The patient may have seizures and become comatose in severe cases. Neurological symptoms vary but generally include blindness in one or both eyes, extreme weakness or paralysis, and poor muscle coordination.

ADEM can be misdiagnosed as multiple sclerosis (MS). However, there are several distinct features that separate these two conditions. The person will have a recent history of a viral illness, such as measles, with a fever and mental status changes that suddenly occur. Children are more often diagnosed with ADEM and rarely diagnosed with MS. ADEM is commonly a single-episode event with a full recovery, whereas such is not the case with MS. MS is an autoimmune disorder that attacks the myelin sheath, usually affects women in their thirties, and is unpredictable. Corticosteroid therapy improves ADEM symptoms, and healing begins within days of treatment. Few patients will have residual neurological deficits or a reoccurrence.

SEVERE COMPLICATIONS OF NATURALLY OCCURRING MEASLES

Most people, including children, recover from measles without serious problems or long-term deficits. However, there are several serious, even fatal, complications with naturally occurring measles. *Encephalitis* is the medical term for inflammation of the brain; symptoms range from mild long-term deficits to life-threatening. One common side effect is seizures. Seizures are an uncontrolled electrical activity of the brain and could lead to a diagnosis of epilepsy. Pneumonia is the most common adverse effect of measles and may result in extensive respiratory deficits. A rare but severe bleeding disorder, ITP is a life-threatening condition that be the result of having measles.

Encephalitis

Encephalitis is the most frequent neurological complication of measles. This condition can occur during a measles infection or as a result of brain inflammation after the illness. The immune system attacks the brain tissue, causing the brain to swell, which puts pressure on the brain tissue and can lead to a headache, photophobia (light sensitivity), and confusion. The neurological status can span from mild confusion and drowsiness to complete unresponsiveness and a comatose state. One to three in a thousand children will develop encephalitis with measles, of whom approximately 15 percent will die. Children who survive infectious encephalitis have a 25 percent probability of a permanent neurological deficit resulting from damage to the neurons (nerve cells) from the infection or the inflammation. There is a wide variation of damage possible, and everyone is affected differently. Impairment may be cognitive, physical, emotional, or behavioral.

Cognitive damage refers to a mental process in the brain, including attention, memory, and language skills. Complex processes such as problem-solving and decision-making may be reduced to the point that daily activities become complicated and impede independent life. Encephalitis may decrease the ability to think and process new information on time due to a lack of concentration. Patients and families are advised to reduce the external stimuli of the afflicted individual and to assist in beginning tasks and completing one task at a time.

Memory deficits are common in patients with encephalitis; they have difficulty processing old and new memories or new events and people. This deficit can be very frustrating to patients and result in aggressive or depressive behavior. Simple everyday tasks like brushing their teeth must be relearned, and the task often needs visual cues. Executive function is impaired whenever cognitive functions are diminished. Executive function is the higher-level cognitive skills, such as planning, inhibition, intuition, and problem-solving. Difficulty in any of these areas impedes a person's ability to accomplish tasks like balancing a checkbook, paying bills, and even having a normal relationship with another person. This disorder reduces the ability to complete tasks and conduct effective time management, all skills required to maintain a job.

A neuropsychological assessment is used to determine the cognitive changes after encephalitis. A rehabilitation plan is a long-term strategy to manage cognitive problems and improve the ability to conduct the activities of everyday living. An even more alarming effect is reduced awareness or insight of those deficits afflicting the sufferer. Older patients are more susceptible to this difficulty because they have some consciousness of having had a previous life that was "normal." The person is unaware of the changes that have occurred in the brain itself. This lack of self-awareness affects their perception of what tasks, such as driving, relationships, and working, have been altered. The person may deny any issues, thereby presenting challenges for their safety and the safety of others.

Confabulation is another memory problem associated with encephalitis and loss of executive function. The person suffering from confabulation has false memories that seem real and also lose the ability to discern the difference between reality and illusion. The person may talk in great detail about a visit they recently had with their parents, providing information on the conversation and the meal they shared, even though the person's parents died several years prior. The memory is real to this person, and they cannot comprehend that this is a false memory. People with this deficit, combined with the inability to identify, plan, and organize high-level cognitive skills, often require twenty-four-hour supervision.

The linguistic difficulties associated with encephalitis further complicate the long-term effects of encephalitis. The problems include an inability to understand what is said, known as *receptive aphasia*, or the inability to comprehend spoken or written words. This disorder causes difficulty learning or following tasks, such as following directions or reading a book. A person with this disorder needs extensive therapy with a speech-language pathologist that is designed to address the specific needs of the person. Another disorder is the inability to express thoughts or needs appropriately. This lack of communication skills, termed *expressive aphasia*, means the person can receive and comprehend speech and reading but is unable to render their thoughts into words that make sense. The person may use disassociated words, known as a *word salad*, such as "Blue cat fly eat." The words are connected but fail to communicate what the person needs or wants. Expressive aphasia results in the inability to ask questions or develop age-appropriate language skills. Speech therapy can assist in improving expressive language deficits like this but require intensive and lengthy treatment plans.

One unusual characteristic associated with encephalitis is prosopagnosia, or face blindness. Prosopagnosia is the inability to recognize faces, even those of close friends and family members. The person may be able to recall the knowledge stored about the individual with some prompts. The ability may return if the person says their name and shares a memory but is not retained. This disorder is rare and associated with other cognitive or visual difficulties.

The most common complaint after encephalitis is extreme fatigue and weakness. This fatigue can be so disabling that simple everyday tasks are overwhelming and require assistance. Other issues include tremors and seizures. Medications are available to help control both but must be continued for life and often have severe side effects. People who have suffered encephalitis may also experience behavioral and emotional changes. Anxiety and depression are common and are managed with antianxiety medications. Disinhibition and emotional regulation are more challenging to accomplish since the person is often unaware of inappropriate behavior and becomes verbally or physically aggressive. Although some antipsychotic medications may diminish the response, they cannot correct the damage to the brain. People with severe encephalitis require continual supervision or may need to reside in a locked unit for their safety.

A rare but progressive and deadly form of encephalitis called *subacute sclerosing panencephalitis* (SSPE) may be seen with measles. Most people diagnosed with SSPE die within three years of diagnosis, while others suffer a rapid disease progression and expire within a few weeks. The symptoms tend to develop approximately ten years after having recovered from measles with no immediate residual issues. The virus remains in the central nervous system and slowly degenerates the myelin sheath of those cells, which assists in the electrical conduction from one nerve cell to another.

The person with SSPE will suddenly and without warning experience bizarre neurological symptoms, such as forgetfulness, aggression, sleeplessness, and hallucinations. The symptoms are considered Stage I of the condition and may last several months, but since the symptoms are vague, the disorder may remain undiagnosed until the onset of Stage II. People diagnosed with SSPE are often misdiagnosed with a psychiatric illness, thereby delaying an appropriate response to the condition. Stage II is marked by loss of motor function, resulting in uncontrolled movements and spasms. Seizures and dementia may be seen in this stage. A lumbar puncture is performed to arrive at the correct diagnosis, as fluid drawn from the measles patient is the gold standard for diagnosing SSPE. Stage III includes the complete loss of muscle control, at which point the person is usually unresponsive. The brain stem is affected during Stage IV, resulting in coma and eventually death. There is no cure or treatment for SSPE. Once the symptoms begin, the disease continues to progress. According to the CDC, 7 to 11 of every 100,000 people who have had measles are at risk of developing SSPE. Children who have had measles at two years of age have been found to have a slightly higher incidence rate for SSPE.

Seizures and Epilepsy

A seizure is the consequence of uncontrolled electrical activity in the brain. It can cause strange movements or sensations and produces changes in the level of consciousness or environmental awareness. Some people having a seizure may exhibit spastic movements of the arms and legs and body stiffness. In contrast, others may stare into space or experience sudden emotional episodes, such as screaming or crying. Most people have no recollection of the attack and are confused once the seizure has passed. Two or more recurring episodes of seizures lead to a diagnosis of epilepsy. Seizures are common with encephalitis in the acute phase and increase the risk of epilepsy. Viral encephalitis is frequently associated with subsequent epilepsy due to the brain area where the seizures begin. Most viral-related episodes start in the frontal or temporal lobes and are associated with a poor prognosis of recovery or management.

Medications known as antiepileptic drugs help control long-term seizures. However, these drugs have considerable side effects, including hair loss, weight gain, irritability in children, and slower reaction times. Children taking antiepileptic drugs may develop bone fragility and reduced attention span. Women planning to become pregnant and taking antiepileptic medications have an increased risk of congenital infant disabilities. Seizures can be controlled by brain surgery, by which the part of the brain that causes the episodes is removed. The surgery has had good results with epileptic children. Another option is a vagal stimulator, which the Epilepsy Foundation describes as a "pacemaker for the brain." The device is implanted in the chest, and a wire is threaded to the vagus nerve in the neck. Once activated, a mild pulsation of electrical energy is sent to the brain by the vagus nerve. This electrical pulsation disrupts abnormal brain activity that generates a seizure.

Children and adults with epilepsy from encephalitis require long-term antiepileptic medications. Children, unfortunately, have difficulty swallowing the pills or are unable to tolerate the side effects. A ketogenic diet is a modality of controlling seizures that has been used since the 1920s for such children. The diet is based on the consumption of high fat and small amounts of protein and carbohydrates. This diet mimics a fasting state by altering the metabolism in its use of fats as a primary energy source. This process results in the liver producing ketone bodies and urinary ketosis. Evidence supports the use of a ketogenic diet to control seizures. However, it is difficult to follow, and many patients are only compliant for a limited time.

Pneumonia

The CDC reports that 50,000 people die from pneumonia each year in the United States, and pneumonia is one of the leading causes of death for children under the age of five worldwide. Pneumonia may lead to severe and long-term complications, the most concerning of which is septic shock. Septic shock results from the infection entering the bloodstream and causing a dramatic drop in blood pressure. Such a drop means the heart cannot pump enough blood to the organs, upon which these vital organs begin to stop functioning correctly and the patient dies. Sepsis often causes kidney damage because of the inadequate blood supply. Some patients may require hemodialysis to remove toxins from the blood that the kidneys typically accomplish when healthy. Most patients recover quickly from kidney damage, but others will require ongoing medical treatment for months.

The onset of septic shock causes the heart to pump faster to compensate for the inadequate blood volume, making the heart work harder. Low blood pressure also results in rapid breathing, a fever, and gastrointestinal disorders. Confusion is an additional symptom that results from inadequate perfusion to the brain. The onset of septic shock requires aggressive treatment with large volumes of intravenous fluids and medications to help shunt the peripheral blood into the body's main organs. The person often experiences respiratory distress and requires mechanical ventilation while the body fights to recover. Sepsis, or septic shock, is the leading cause of death for patients admitted into an intensive care unit for an issue unrelated to the heart.

Pneumonia may cause pockets of infection in the lungs, called *lung abscesses*, that require aggressive antibiotic treatment. The condition and antibiotic therapy can decrease the ability of the body to fight other infections and weaken the immune system. Most patients will have a high fever that spikes at night and a productive cough. They will require assistance with daily living activities, such as bathing, brushing their teeth, and getting dressed. Nutritional support is beneficial to increase strength and overall health.

The outer lining of the lungs, called the *pleura*, helps the lungs move while breathing, but with pneumonia, the pleura swells and causes sharp pain with each breath. The pleura space can also fill with fluid; this condition, preventable by intervention, is called a *pleural effusion*. The pleura space can get infected; the collection of pus is termed *empyema*. Respiratory intervention and antibiotics that are effective against the specific infection of the patient must be implemented to combat empyema.

Respiratory failure is possible for patients with severe pneumonia, as the ability of the blood to transfer oxygen and carbon dioxide in the blood is impeded. When the body cannot get enough oxygen, a person will feel like they cannot get enough air; they will breathe faster, become anxious, and lose consciousness—resulting in a severe condition requiring hospitalization and supplemental oxygen or mechanical ventilation. The patient's underlying medical conditions dictate whether this could lead to a lengthy recovery period and permanent respiratory difficulties.

The heart may be affected permanently by pneumonia, as the CDC reports that 20 percent of patients hospitalized with pneumonia will develop heart failure. Heart failure is the inability of the heart to pump blood efficiently. The reason could be the stress of having pneumonia or the result of the inflammatory process. The condition is usually chronic and progressive and will require medications and lifestyle changes to control. Patients with heart failure are often hospitalized from exacerbations of the situation. An article by Duflos et al. published in *Scientific Reports* (2020) followed 223 patients with heart failure and found that hospitalization was required in approximately 60 percent of all such patients during one year.

Long-Term Complications from Naturally Occurring Measles

Measles may also cause an illness many years after the infection. Ten to twenty years after surviving measles, the infection can lead to a rare but fatal form of encephalitis, known as subacute sclerosing panencephalitis (SSPE). The virus remains in the central nervous system and slowly degenerates the myelin sheathing of the nerve cells. The myelin sheath assists the electrical conduction from one nerve cell to another. Children with SSPE gradually decline in cognitive function and display inappropriate behavior, which may lead them to be misdiagnosed with a psychiatric disorder. New-onset seizures prompt a lumbar puncture to evaluate the cerebral spinal fluid. A definitive diagnosis of SSPE is made if the results of this procedure indicate measles in the fluid.

How measles persists in the brain for years is unknown. Some countries report geographic clustering of SSPE and rural areas have a higher incidence rate. Two studies from the early 1900s found that children near birds have an increased incidence of SSPE. According to the CDC, research suggests an environmental factor, but nothing has been definitively identified. This condition is 100 percent fatal; those afflicted will gradually deteriorate until they become comatose and die.

Neurological Disorders from Naturally Occurring Measles

The National Institute of Neurological Disorders and Stroke (NINDS) and the National Institutes of Health (NIH) collaboratively research neurological disorders that arise from measles. Several researchers conducting studies are seeking answers on why the immune system attacks the insulating substance called *myelin*. Other researchers are in quest of procedures to repair the myelin sheath to allow for optimal nerve conduction. Research currently focuses on the oligodendrocyte cells that make up the myelin sheath surrounding the neuronal axons. Funding by the NINDS and NIH supports research on cellular functions that control the maturation and regeneration of myelin. Other researchers look to the interventions that can reduce damage from demyelination. These scientists are hopeful that research on the Brahma-related gene 1 (Brg1) will clarify the molecular functions of the central nervous system myelination and remyelination. They hope to develop a chemical compound that mimics the Brg1 and enhances remyelination activities.

7

Effects on Family and Friends

Measles affects the patient directly, but it indirectly impacts family, friends and finances. A noticeable impact is that the patient must isolate to prevent others from being exposed to measles, but isolation has less obvious negative consequences. Isolation increases the release of stress hormones, which creates a systemic inflammatory response. The effects are equally felt by children and adults. Family dynamics must adapt to the isolation and may result in detrimental results—emotional and financial. Children are especially vulnerable to isolation, even for short periods. Financially, contracting measles or caring for a child with measles requires missing work and paying for medical expenses. On a broader scope, communities bear the financial burden of paying for the human resources needed to monitor and implement vaccination campaigns.

ISOLATION DURING THE CONTAGIOUS PERIOD

Isolation is the state of being separated—either forced or voluntarily—from others. Long-term isolation results in acute loneliness, which has been associated with higher levels of the stress-related hormone cortisol. Drs. Leah Doane and Emma Adam researched the association between isolation (loneliness) and cortisol levels for their article "Loneliness and Cortisol: Momentary, Day-to-Day, and Trait Associations," published in

Psychoneuroendocrinology (2010). The physicians sought to link the patho-physiological factors of the stress-induced release of cortisol and self-reported chronic feelings of loneliness. They found that cortisol levels in the blood were elevated in all participants who reported feeling isolated, even for short periods.

According to the article "Feel Lonely? There Are 4 Types of Loneliness. Here's How to Beat Them" (Biddlecombe, 2018), there are four distinct types of loneliness: emotional, situational, social, and chronic. *Emotional loneliness* comes from within a person, an intrinsic disconnect. This form of loneliness has various causes, including experiences, background, and personal dissatisfaction. Therapy with a mental health counselor or psychologist often helps to identify the issues and develop a resolution plan. *Situational loneliness* stems from circumstances that make relationships difficult. This form of isolation may result from starting a new job or moving to a new city. The best approach to resolving situational loneliness is actively seeking new social connections and realizing that this will take time. To resolve situational loneliness requires honest self-reflection and working with professional help.

Being shy, socially awkward, or having low self-esteem is usually the cause of social loneliness. *Social loneliness* is experienced by people who lack social contact or interactions with others. It is a lack of connection. You can live alone but have adequate social interaction. You can also live with others but feel isolated. The U.S. Department of Health and Human Services states that all people need social connection to survive, especially during an illness. *Chronic loneliness* may lead to depression, illness, and thoughts of suicide. Identifying the reason for loneliness is essential to developing a plan of treatment. A visit to a general practitioner or counseling service and having a frank discussion on the issue can begin the healing process. Medications may be needed to help overcome the depressive feelings.

For most people, having measles is a short-term episodic event but may cause social and situational loneliness. The feelings should resolve when the person heals from measles and can begin to socialize again. If measles is severe and requires an extended recovery period, the loneliness may worsen and lead to depression. Severe complications, such as pneumonia or encephalitis, may result in extreme depression from chronic loneliness. A study published in the *Community Mental Health Journal* (2019) found a significant increase of depression and suicidal ideation with patients that had a chronic illness with poor quality of life and a lack of family support. The article, titled "Suicide Risk and Depression in Individuals with Chronic Illness," used the Beck Depression Scale and found a significant positive relationship between chronic illness and poor mental health.

Humans were not designed to be isolated creatures and need interaction with others to feel a sense of belonging. The isolation required of a person with measles alters the ability to be with others. A person diagnosed with measles or any other contagious disease should immediately self-isolate to reduce the risk of exposing unvaccinated people to the infection. Still, it is essential to recognize that this isolation has detrimental consequences for children and adults that may not be immediately evident.

Vulnerable Children

Vulnerable children may be isolated to prevent their risk of exposure to measles. Children in this population include those with asthma, cancer, and type 1 diabetes and the immunocompromised. Children diagnosed with cancer have a much greater probability of getting infected with measles, resulting in severe complications or death. This increased risk occurs even if the child has had the two-dose MMR vaccination. The barrage of medications given to children with cancer prevents the correct functioning of the immune system. Chemotherapy eradicates the cancer cells, but it also attacks the memory of the immune system such that it does not recognize the intrusion of pathogens such as measles, leaving them to attack healthy cells in the body.

The most common form of childhood cancer is leukemia, which accounts for one out of three childhood cancers, according to the American Cancer Society (2019). Treatment for leukemia is a two or three year treatment plan. During that time, it severely diminishes the immune system's ability to function during this period and up to six months after treatment has ended, and it impedes the body's ability to fight any infections. Most children can usually deal with common colds and benign viruses, but exposure to severe illnesses, such as measles, would overwhelm a compromised immune system. Due to the fragile immune system of a person undergoing chemotherapy, getting vaccinated or revaccinated is not an option until several months after the completion of treatment.

A devastating measles outbreak in New Zealand from 2010 to 2011 had a death rate of 50 percent among immunocompromised children; the majority of this population were children diagnosed with cancer and undergoing chemotherapy. Previous immunizations for all childhood illnesses only partially protect these children from childhood illnesses, and in some cases, they do not protect them at all. The Ministry of Health for New Zealand published the *Protecting Children with Cancer from Measles* pamphlet in 2012 to address concerns about isolating vulnerable children and their families during a measles outbreak. When the measles outbreak began in New Zealand, a ten-year-old child named Kelcey Roberts had just completed her last chemotherapy for acute lymphoblastic leukemia. The administration at the school that Kelcey attended immediately notified her parents. Kelcey stopped attending school because several students were unvaccinated. The risk of exposure was too significant for Kelcey to have a potential measles exposure, and she was isolated. Kelcey and her entire family felt the effects of isolation. All social activities were canceled, and the family banned all nonfamilial children from entering the house. Tracey Roberts, Kelcey's mother, said her daughter did not understand why being around unvaccinated children was an issue. Kelcey was a typical adolescent who enjoyed social activities with others her age. However, her parents understood the risks. Just leaving the house and visiting a fast-food restaurant could expose their daughter to measles. The risk of exposure came from other children and contaminated surfaces.

Another child, Shauna Manning, was diagnosed with leukemia during the summer before entering kindergarten. Shauna was isolated from other children and even her relatives that lived nearby for the next thirteen months. The family planned to keep Shauna isolated for at least a year to allow her immune system to recover from the chemotherapy, after which Shauna could be reimmunized for measles and hopefully remain healthy. The entire family was restricted in their social activities during this period of isolation because of Shauna's fragile immune system.

Many times, the isolation can significantly affect the psychological development of children. The parents of Cooper, a twenty-month-old toddler, expressed great concern after their son was diagnosed with acute lymphoblastic leukemia. The leukemia was aggressive, and his treatment plan extended for over three years. Cooper was isolated from contact with other children and developed a withdrawn attitude toward other people. His parents were most concerned about his increased anxiety around all young children, even children who were family members and considered safe.

Physical isolation is required when a child or adult is contagious or vulnerable to being exposed to measles. However, physical isolation also affects social development because it is central to the development of human beings. This behavior includes feelings and thoughts influenced by interactions with others and is vital for children who must learn these socialization skills. When children are deprived of social interactions, their mental health and development is hindered.

Dr. Caspi and associates followed an entire birth cohort of 1,037 children to age 26 years. The researchers measured social isolation during childhood and those diagnosed with adult cardiovascular disease and posted their findings in the *Archives of Pediatric Adolescent Medicine* (2006). Multifactorial risk factors such as weight, blood pressure, and cholesterol were gathered for the study but not used to analyze the risk factors in the study. The researchers concluded that loneliness from social isolation compromises a person's health, rendering them especially vulnerable to coronary artery disease later in life. The study measured isolation using the Rutter Child Scales, then the Wechsler Intelligence Scales for Children was subsequently administered. The statistical analysis revealed a direct correlation between social isolation in childhood and adult cardiovascular risk factors.

This study was the catalyst for the National Child Development Study (2014) by Drs. Rebecca Lacey, Meena Kumari, and Mel Bartley, which evaluated the correlation of childhood social isolation between C-reactive protein (CRP) and psychological distress and health behaviors in adulthood. CRP is made in the liver and released into the bloodstream in response to inflammation. Inflammation is the body's response to fighting infections, injuries, and toxins that could cause harm. The release of the chemicals triggers a reaction from the immune system.

The researchers hypothesized that social isolation in childhood increased the risk of inflammation across the individual's life span. Substantial research has linked childhood isolation with alcoholism, drug abuse, and depression. Not only did the study reveal that isolated children had a higher level of CRP, but it also led the researchers to conclude that such children also exhibited psychological distress, obesity, and addictive behaviors such as smoking and alcohol.

FINANCIAL IMPACT

Measles has a deleterious financial impact on the patient, family, and community. The economic impact of measles for a typical family in the United States can be devastating. The average length of illness is fourteen days, meaning that the parent(s) of a child with measles may be out of work during this period to provide care in isolation. The median household income for a family of four with two working parents who have a high school education is $63,179, according to the U.S. Census Bureau of 2018. Two weeks of missing work decreases this annual income by approximately $2,632.00, a financial challenge for most families. The matter is even more dire for single parents, most of whom are women. The median income for a family led by a single mother was approximately $45,128 in 2018. More than ten million low-income families in the United States have one or more children; about four million of these families are led by single mothers. Many of these single parents have no college education and work jobs in the restaurant or hospitality industry. Single mothers in this income bracket make less than a $1,000 per week for food, shelter, and clothing. Ten to fourteen days of lost work could cause them to lose their home or not have money for food or medicine.

Communities in the United States also feel the financial burden of measles. According to the Centers for Disease Control and Prevention (CDC), the cost of public health officials responding to a single measles case range from $5,655 to $181,679. Predominate cost expenditures include personnel to conduct contact tracing. The additional cost is the postexposure prophylaxis (PEP) and the coordination of local, state, and, possibly, international response efforts. One Colorado measles case in 2016 involved a boy with a cough, coryza, and conjunctivitis for three days. Four days later, the maculopapular rash appeared on his head and spread down to cover the torso and legs. The child had returned from a visit to India a few weeks prior and had not received the MMR vaccine. He was placed in airborne isolation upon admission to the local hospital. The period of infectivity is at least eight days: four days before the appearance of the rash and four days after the rash onset. During those eight days, the child had exposed people at the apartment building where he lived, the grocery store, several retail stores, and a fast-food restaurant. The local health department interviewed 311 people who were potentially exposed. Of those, 31 susceptible contacts received PEP, 9 additional contacts received the MMR vaccine, and 22 received immunoglobin therapy. The cost for this public health surveillance that originated with a single case of measles was $49,769.

Another case was a thirty-three-year-old man who traveled to Thailand, who upon returning to the United States developed a fever and rash. The gentleman was hospitalized, where he tested positive for measles. During the infectious period, he had visited seventeen businesses and two separate health-care facilities. Approximately 250 contacts were interviewed, and 232 of these were considered potentially exposed. Only three contacts were unimmunized, and all three were quarantined. The cost for this measles case spanned three public health agencies and the two health-care facilities using 435 personnel hours for a cost of over $18,000.

Measles killed over 200,000 people globally in 2019; this was a twenty-three-year high. The measles cases cost a staggering $42 million based on the statistical data collected by Dr. Jamison Pike, a health economist with the CDC's National Center for Immunization and Respiratory Diseases. Dr. Pike and his colleagues (2020) determined that the eleven outbreaks' overall median cost was $152 300, with a daily cost of over $10,000. The cost does not represent the direct medical cost or the costs associated with missing work. Incorporating this could quickly raise the yearly cost to over $50 million.

In 2019, the World Health Organization (WHO) conducted a retrospective study on the economic burden of measles in the small country of Romania. Romania had a low vaccination rate and experienced a significant outbreak from 2011 to 2012. The costs included in the report were household, health-care provider, and national outbreak response costs. The direct and indirect household costs showed that most of the money was spent on medication, transportation, and missed work. Most families reported an average of twelve days of lost workdays, with the most being sixty-eight. During this outbreak, over $3 million was disbursed to health-care providers. Costs for surveillance and diagnostic testing exceeded $1 million. The economic burden of addressing current measles cases impedes the ability to afford an effective vaccination campaign.

Globally, the message from the WHO is that measles is a vaccine-preventable disease "that can lead to long-term health complication and even death; we cannot afford to be complacent," according to Zsuzsanna Jakab, the WHO regional director for Europe (WHO, 2013). The cost of measles cases is high globally, but it is highest in developing countries. The infrastructure of developing countries is strained between caring for those who have naturally acquired measles and the costs associated with vaccinating the people. The future of measles is frightening; an upswing in measles cases was reported in 2019 across the world, according to the American Red Cross, the CDC, the WHO, and the Pan American Health Organization (PAHO). All of these global organizations have partnered to increase vaccination. The cost of battling a preventable disease with a vaccine costing less than two dollars is too high.

8

Prevention

This chapter begins by defining how the immune system protects the body against pathogens that cause illness. With an understanding of the immune system, how the measles, mumps, and rubella vaccine (MMR) offers protection is then discussed. Exposure to measles can occur via physical contact, airborne droplets, or contaminated surfaces, and all these routes are thoroughly reviewed. One way to prevent the spread of measles is through isolation; however, this is difficult in today's mobile society. Before traveling, a titer (blood test) can determine whether a person has antibodies against measles or needs a booster shot of the measles vaccine. The vaccine provides 97 percent protection from acquiring the naturally occurring measles. Some people that are immunocompromised or allergic to a vaccine ingredient are not able to be vaccinated. Other less effective methods can reduce exposure to measles for this population.

THE IMMUNE SYSTEM

The immune system is the body's protection against attacks by germs and keeps the body healthy. The purpose of the immune system is to distinguish between a foreign particle and the self. *Self* refers to all particles that are part of the body, including cells and tissues. When the immune system is working correctly, particles of the self are protected. The *nonself* particles are not part of the body and are potentially harmful. These foreign bodies can be bacteria, viruses, or parasites and produce proteins called *antigens* that the body recognizes as damaging. Communication of the need to respond to an antigen comes through *cytokines*. Cytokines are the traffic cops of the immune system; they tell the immune system where to go within the body.

Innate Immunity

The immune system contains three components: innate, adaptive, and passive immunity. The three separate components of the immune system work independently and collaboratively. The *innate* component is naturally acquired immunity or general protection, including a physical barrier to germs to prevent entrance into the body. An excellent example of this is the skin, which acts as a barrier against germs entering the body. Innate immunity is also a defense mechanism to prevent germ invasions from sources such as secretions and saliva. General innate immune responses, such as inflammation, are considered a part of the natural immune system by responding to anything foreign (nonself). It is immediately activated upon recognition of a foreign pathogen.

There are several cells within the innate immune system with specific roles in defending the body from infections. *Leukocytes* (white blood cells) are critical to an effective immune system. A *phagocyte* is a type of leukocyte that consumes invading organisms. Phagocytes circulate within the body, ready to attack and destroy, and are commonly called the security guards of the immune system. However, phagocytes are limited to traveling within the confines of the circulatory system. *Macrophages*, a special type of phagocyte, can exit the circulatory system and seek out pathogens. They release cytokines once a pathogen has been located to recruit other cells to destroy the invading germs. *Mast cells* defend against pathogens by starting the inflammatory cascade, which begins with releasing histamine and cytokines. Histamine causes blood vessels to dilate; thus, additional blood will flow into the area. Cytokines message other cells to begin the attack on the pathogen. Several other specialized cells assist in the immune system. The *neutrophil* cell is a phagocyte that explicitly attacks bacteria. A complete blood count (CBC) is a blood test that reveals the number of phagocytes, which helps the physician develop a plan of treatment that will assist in destroying unwelcome germs.

Complement System

The *complement system* works synergistically with the innate immune system as a variety of proteins with specialized jobs. *Opsonization* tags infected cells and identifies the pathogens that have the same antigens. *Chemotaxis* is a chemical signal for macrophages to begin the destruction process. Cell *lysis* destroys the pathogens' cell membranes by puncturing them, thereby weakening their ability to proliferate and killing the cell. *Agglutination* binds pathogens together, allowing the immune system to efficiently attack and destroy the pathogen.

Adaptive Immune System

The innate immune system is the initial response to a pathogen, but sometimes it is not enough to destroy the invader. When that happens, an *adaptive* immune system must be recruited. The adaptive immune system uses only two specialized cells: the *B lymphocyte*, or B cell, and the *T lymphocyte*, or T cell. *Lymphocytes* create a memory of the invaders and seek them out for destruction. Both cells develop in the bone marrow, and some of them remain in the marrow and mature into the B cells, which make antibodies. The B lymphocyte and T lymphocyte cells are the military system for the body. B lymphocytes are the intelligence system, as they seek out a target (antigen). Once the B lymphocytes identify an invader, they create antibodies as a memory. Then they call upon the T lymphocytes, as the soldiers of the immune system, to attack. They destroy the invaders that the B lymphocytes have identified as nonself.

Antibodies remain within the immune system, ready to fight these antigens if they enter the body again. This is the premise for vaccines that introduce an antigen to the body but do not make the person ill. The immune system recognizes the antigen and makes antibodies to protect the person from a future attack. B lymphocytes recognize and seek out the antigen within the body but cannot destroy it. That is the job of the soldiers, the T lymphocytes. Known as the "killer cells," these cells signal the phagocytes to consume the invaders.

Passive Immunity

Passive immunity happens when a person is given antibodies to a disease instead of producing them with their own immune system. Newborn babies obtain passive immunity from their mothers through the placenta. Antibodies are also received by the infant in breast milk or given via an injection of gamma globulin. Infants have passive immunity against measles if their mother is immune. The antibodies gradually disappear by six months of age and are completely gone at one year.

Immunological Memory

Long-lasting protection from many infections is available because the immune system learns and remembers pathogens, a condition known as *immunological memory*. This memory enables the body to make antibodies against a variety of pathogens. This protection is where the MMR vaccine enters the concept of immune memory, as it contains an attenuated (weakened) virus of measles, mumps, and rubella. The virus cannot cause an active infection but mimics the virus closely enough to initiate an immune response. The vaccine exposes the body to the antigen. Afterward, the immune system produces an antibody to the virus and creates a memory without actually getting ill. This process is why vaccines are a safe and effective method for controlling a contagious virus like measles.

Immune Amnesia

Measles is directly responsible for over 100,000 yearly deaths. Its association with increased morbidity and mortality years after the illness is questioned by scientists and epidemiologists. Several studies have suggested a connection between how measles infects the immune cells and long-term immune suppression. Scientists have termed this phenomenon *immune amnesia*, which can increase the risk of diseases and infections for years. Given the resurgence of this disease, scientists must understand how measles affects the immune system long term to be able to mitigate the reaction.

Dr. Michael Mina was the lead researcher for a 2019 study that involved a Dutch community with low vaccination rates. This community was currently having a measles outbreak and provided the perfect scenario to evaluate immune suppression associated with wild-type measles and children who had received the MMR vaccine. A total of seventy-seven unimmunized participants enrolled in the study. The children had blood drawn for testing using VirScan, a laboratory test that tracks measles antibodies before being exposed to measles or receiving the MMR vaccine. Testing was conducted at the beginning of the study, two months postexposure, and one year later.

The cumulative results of the study supported the theory of immune amnesia after measles diagnosis. The antibody results showed a potential vulnerability of the immune system to respond to future infections. Past studies have indicated a drop of 5–10 percent of antibodies in people suffering from measles: However, using VirScan's new technology, children with a mild case of measles lost 33 percent of their immune capability, and with severe measles, the loss was in the 40 percent range.

Dr. Mina compared the loss to damage to the immune system by the human immunodeficiency virus (HIV), which is a disease that interferes with the ability of the body to respond to infections. The immunological memory destroyed by untreated HIV takes approximately five years, but measles can generate the same response as a measles infection. The catch in this path is that the immune system of a person with measles can be regenerated, whereas HIV patients cannot regain the functionality of their immune system by any means known to date. The time frame for rebuilding the immune system and recovering the antibody memory lost with immune amnesia takes two to three years. During this time, children are especially highly vulnerable to a variety of infections and illnesses.

Dr. V. Petrova and associates published a study titled "Incomplete Genetic Reconstitution of B Cell Pools Contributes to Prolonged Immunosuppression after Measles" in *Science Immunology* (2019) on the effect of measles and a specific immune system component. B lymphocytes, or B cells, are a type of white blood cell produced in the bone marrow; they migrate to lymph tissues throughout the body for maturation. Once mature, these cells have a Y-shaped protein called *antibodies*. If the antibodies recognize any pathogen as foreign, a complex chain of events begins in the immune system. Foreign particles are investigated, and it is determined whether they are harmful. If the particles are dangerous, antibodies lock on to the surface of specific pathogens and recruit other cells in the immune system to destroy all pathogen elements.

These European researchers specifically designed their study to determine how measles infection affects B cells' reconstitution and suppression within the immune system. A total of twenty-three Dutch children participated in the study. The researchers examined B cell receptor sequencing before and after participants had been diagnosed with measles. B cells were found to be immunologically immature after measles, meaning that they were slower to mature into cells that could actively participate in identifying foreign particles or infections. The memory cells associated with B cells were depleted based on the levels before having measles, which put a person at an increased risk for severe complications from infections. This study was similar to the one conducted by Dr. Michael Mina and associates. Both studies indicate there appears to be a lengthy recovery period of the immune system after a measles infection.

MEASLES, MUMPS, AND RUBELLA VACCINE

The vaccine antigens are primarily derived from the Edmonston strain in the United States, but non-Edmonston strains are available in other countries. Excipients (inactive substances) in vaccines are minute ingredients serving a specific purpose, such as acting preservatives, stabilizers, or antibiotics. Neomycin is the most common antibiotic used in the MMR vaccine. Stabilizers in this antibiotic include sorbitol or gelatin. Gelatin is a protein derived from boiling skin or connective tissue, and all gelatin used in vaccines originates from porcine (pig) sources. Since many religions oppose pork consumption, sorbitol is an alternative stabilizer naturally produced in the body and found in many berries and fruits. The virus used for the vaccine (with either gelatin or sorbitol stabilizer) is grown in chick embryo cells or human diploid cells in sterile and controlled environments.

The MMR vaccine protects against measles, mumps, and rubella (German measles). The initial dose is scheduled for children to receive between nine and fifteen months of age, which provides a 90 percent protection rate. The second dose is given between fifteen months and six years of age, providing a 97 percent protection rate against measles, 88 percent for mumps, and 97 percent against rubella. The vaccine dose is in 0.5 milliliters of liquid given via a subcutaneous injection. The vaccine is effective for all children and people without evidence of immunity according to the Centers for Disease Control and Prevention (CDC) and the World Health Organization (WHO). It is recommended that those who are unimmunized and exposed to measles receive one dose of the vaccine within seventy-two hours of exposure.

The MMR vaccine is a live-attenuated (weakened) form of the three infections and is safe when administered with other vaccines, such as tetanus, diphtheria, and pertussis (Tdap). Many people receive the vaccine without side effects, while others experience mild complications that do not require any treatment. The most common side effect is pain or redness at the injection site or a slight fever. Only one in one million vaccine recipients will have a severe allergic reaction or anaphylactic shock to a vaccine component, the vaccine itself, the rubber used in the stopper, or a preservative. Older women have an increased non-life-threatening reaction of joint pain or arthritis, which can be acute or chronic. The Food and Drug Administration (FDA) added two rare adverse reactions to the vaccination label in 2014: transverse myelitis and acute disseminated encephalomyelitis (ADEM).

Only 3 out of 100 people will not serum convert with the two-dose vaccination and contract the infection when exposed. Scientists cannot identify the exact reasons but hypothesize that there is a deficit within the immune system or that the ability to fight the disease decreases with age or comorbidities. The symptoms in such cases are less severe and are quick to dissipate. The immunization will reduce the risk of spreading the infection to others.

LIMITING EXPOSURE

Children under the age of five are especially susceptible to being exposed to measles through physical contact. They play near one another and often do not practice safe hygiene. Their focus is on the activity during play, and they often neglect to cover their mouth or turn their head when they sneeze or cough. Young children can be taught the "vampire" cough as good practice by covering the mouth with the arm's inside area with the elbow pointing out. This method is easy to teach and a better strategy than using their hands because hands can further spread germs unless washed immediately afterward. Older children can understand and practice the more complex procedures to limit exposure through physical contact, namely wearing a mask in public, not touching the face, and good handwashing.

Airborne exposure is an additional way that a person can be exposed to measles. Even with casual or transient contact, the airspace of an infected person is a danger zone. The aerosolized droplets released from talking, sneezing, or coughing are suspended in the air well after they are expelled—even after the infected person has left the area for up to two hours! One reason that measles is so contagious is that the virus can live suspended in the air for such a long period. The risk of airborne exposure increases in small enclosed areas, such as school classrooms, offices, buses, and airplanes. The virus can infect another person without any knowledge of how it occurred. Scientists have deduced that there are minimal actions available that can reduce airborne exposure. However, sunlight can reduce the life span of airborne measles from two hours to two minutes. Heat, an acidic pH, and the enzyme trypsin, which is found in the small intestine, can reduce or kill the virus; this process is discussed in detail in chapter 3.

The third method of viral transmission is the most pervasive. Hard surfaces can harbor the active contagion for approximately two hours because such characters allow the fine mist of a cough or sneeze to remain unabsorbed. When a person with measles has a conversation, coughs, or sneezes, the mist is propelled approximately six feet in an arc-like trajectory. The falling particles land on surrounding hard surfaces and can effectively infect another person who comes in contact with that surface by touching it with a hand and then touching the face without washing their hands. Desks, doorknobs, toys, and seats are just a few of the items commonly found to harbor the active measles virus. Exposure can be limited by consistently cleaning hard surfaces within the home using soap or disinfectants. Using a paper towel or tissue to open doors will also assist in decreasing exposure. The most effective method of exposure reduction is also the least expensive; effective handwashing is the best option.

Isolation

The only two methods of effectively preventing measles are the MMR vaccine and isolation from any known person or situation. To avoid exposure, the unvaccinated person would have to avoid all physical contact with any other unvaccinated person for their entire lifetime. Travel would be minimal, and the only permissible movement would occur within a protected environment. Additionally, the airspace would have to be protected from potential contagions, a condition of isolation that would require extreme diligence as the virus can remain suspended in the air for up to two hours.

Isolation is not a feasible option for today's society; even cultures that live in a self-contained environment, such as the Amish, risk exposure. The Amish are a Christian sect from the Swiss Anabaptist movement. They practice group solidarity and reject all modern conveniences. Their religious beliefs do not expressly oppose vaccines, but they strictly limit interaction with preventive health care outside their community. Vaccinations are not encouraged, which contributes to the low vaccination rates among this population. When an outbreak occurs, the virus runs rampant through Amish community members who are unvaccinated.

This scenario happened in Ohio when two Amish men traveled to the Philippines as mission relief workers for the massive typhoon in 2014. The Philippines was already suffering a measles outbreak at this time, with over 21,000 cases and more than 100 deaths just before the storm struck. The two unvaccinated men returned to the United States unknowingly infected with measles. After returning to their Amish community—the members of which were unvaccinated or only partially protected—there were over 300 cases of measles reported and over 100 deaths. The transmission was rampant and affected over 68 percent of the Amish households in nine counties. This strain of measles was genotype D9, which was the same strain currently affecting the Philippines. Public officials quickly began a vaccination campaign to inoculate over 10,000 people. Containment efforts were also implemented to isolate anyone with measles symptoms (rash and fever) and quarantine immunocompromised people.

Relying on isolation to prevent a measles outbreak would require extreme diligence and avoidance of anyone who is sick, whether or not they show any symptoms. Measles can be contagious before the appearance of the classic rash; the insipid nature of the symptoms makes avoiding measles difficult to impossible. The WHO classifies measles as a febrile rash illness. The incubation period for measles is between ten and fourteen days but can be seven to twenty-three days from exposure to symptom onset. The prodromal (initial) phase begins with malaise and fever, followed by a cough, conjunctivitis (inflamed eyes), and coryza (runny nose).

The hallmark maculopapular rash presents two to four days after the initial symptoms or ten to twelve days after exposure. The rash may appear as early as seven days and as long as twenty-one days from the time of exposure. Many factors affect the incubation period, including the overall health status and age of the exposed individual.

Any person with a cough, runny nose, and itchy eyes from allergies mimics the symptoms of measles, making isolation ineffective in preventing exposure to measles. The initial symptoms are too generic to assess the risk accurately. Some safeguards can limit exposure for populations that are unable to be vaccinated. This tactic includes avoiding interaction with all known unvaccinated people; this includes members of any vaccine-hesitant religious organizations and anyone entirely against vaccination. It is generally easy to identify vaccine-hesitant religious organizations through a quick internet search, but individual opinions are more difficult to ascertain. The parent of an immunocompromised child should know that becoming infected with this virus could be life-threatening and must speak out as an advocate for their child. Parents of such children should limit time spent with all other children in social settings and have a frank conversation with the child's pediatrician.

PRECAUTIONS FOR INTERNATIONAL TRAVEL

Federal officials are evaluating the potential of banning persons with active symptoms from flying to combat the potential spread of measles during travel. There have also been conversations with the Department of Homeland Security about creating a public do-not-board list for travelers with a probability of measles. The do-not-board list began in 2007 to block a man with drug-resistant tuberculosis from flying to Europe. Government officials have since enforced the policy for restricting persons with active measles cases from entering the United States.

All international travelers in individual and group arrangements should be sure all group members have been protected against measles, regardless of the destination. Those who do not have evidence of immunity are at risk for exposure because of the current global outbreaks. Proof of immunity includes written documentation from a health-care provider, a positive titer (blood test), or birth before 1957 in the United States. Without this evidence, the best protection is receiving the two-dose vaccination at least two weeks before traveling and thirty days apart. If it is not feasible to obtain the two doses, taking one dose of the MMR vaccine is prudent.

Measles is still a common illness in many European countries, the Middle East, Africa, and Asia. Other tourist destinations are currently experiencing an outbreak, including Thailand, Vietnam, Japan, and the

Philippines. Over 100,000 people die from measles each year throughout the world. Two out of three unvaccinated travelers are Americans, who can spread the disease while traveling internationally and bring measles back to the United States and initiate an outbreak. Measles is so contagious that 90 percent of unvaccinated people will become infected in close contact with an infectious individual.

The CDC provides a web-based assessment tool from their home page at cdc.gov. for people planning international travel. The instrument adapts to the participant's responses to approximately ten questions, beginning with "Are you traveling internationally?" The next question asks whether the participant was born before 1957. Citizens of the United States born before this year are considered protected against measles. However, this does not exclude the need to receive the MMR vaccine booster when traveling to countries with a current outbreak or high case numbers. Travelers who are less than one year of age or who have no record of receiving the two-dose MMR vaccine are strongly encouraged to get vaccinated. The site explains that there is no harm in getting revaccinated or receiving additional MMR vaccine doses.

Any traveler on long international flights might be sitting near someone with measles. In 2018, over eighty U.S. flights were confirmed to have had at least one contagious person on board. That same year, a fifteen-year-old boy visited England and returned with measles as a souvenir. The virus spread to a sixteen-year-old during a scouting event, who then shared the illness with two other teenagers and adults. The teenager also exposed a seven-year-old who became infected at a tutoring center, and his four-year-old brother also contracted the virus. A total of seven confirmed measles cases were attributed to the unvaccinated fifteen-year-old who visited England over a month before. The outbreak was quickly contained due to the rapid notification and the initiation of contact tracing by public health officials. In another incident, in February 2019, a passenger returning from a business trip in Asia infected two passengers, one adult and one child. A spokesperson for the San Francisco Health Department, Rachael Kagan, said that this was the city's first confirmed case since 2013.

A nineteen-month-old toddler bound for India was waiting in the Chicago airport within the same boarding area as a man from Minnesota who was positive for measles. They were not on the same flight; however, the two had the same measles genotype. It indicated a direct link from the Minnesota resident to the young child. The CDC investigation concluded that the transmission probably occurred through airborne exposure or a contaminated hard surface at the boarding gate. Remember, the virus can travel several feet via cough or sneeze, and it can live for up to two hours on a hard surface.

The issue of unvaccinated travelers spreading measles continues to affect travel. A toddler exposed travelers to measles at O'Hare International Airport in November 2020. Chicago public health officials had confirmed that an unvaccinated thirteen-month-old child returning on an international flight was contagious. The toddler traveled through two separate terminals over three hours. The exposure was sent to all known contacts and provided to the general public via local television stations and news outlets.

MEASLES TITER TEST

Vaccines initiate a variety of antibodies. A titer test determines seropositivity based on the selective antibody concentrations found in the blood. The results are based on positive, negative, or equivocal antibody levels for various infectious diseases and are usually available in three to four days. A positive result indicates that the individual has been exposed to measles through natural exposure to a contagious individual or has received the vaccine. The results specify the presence of the IgG antibodies, which occur through an infection (measles) or immunization. Those who receive positive titer results can be considered immune to measles.

A low or negative titer represents minimal antibodies present in the blood. Low titers mean that the person could get measles and is not immune. A negative titer indicates that the person has no immunity against measles and should be vaccinated. As a person ages, the titer levels may decrease, suggesting that the person needs an MMR booster. Occasionally, postimmunization antibodies are suboptimal, but the person is probably immune.

An equivocal serum test means that the results are indeterminate. The patient may or may not be immune to the virus, but the results cannot be conclusive. As the results are inconclusive, the person should receive the two-dose MMR vaccine. The reason for equivocal results is unknown, but most scientists agree that the person must show positive serum conversion to be protected from measles.

This assumption is not the case for health-care providers. A health-care provider with written documentation of the two-dose MMR vaccine and a measles titer result that is equivocal or negative is not recommended to be revaccinated. The scientific community presumes immunity, and the vaccination supersedes any serological testing. Anyone with documented MMR vaccination does not need to have a titer drawn based on the WHO's guidelines. However, health-care workers with a positive titer are considered fully protected for life, even if the vaccination is undocumented. If the person chooses revaccination or a booster, there is no known risk of receiving additional MMR vaccinations.

Alternatively, some health-care organizations suggest that individuals receive an MMR booster and skip getting a titer drawn during measles outbreaks. These organizations cite the following four reasons: (1) The titer requires an order from a physician, a visit to a laboratory, and waiting for the results. (2) The test results are costly. Most insurance companies have copays for laboratory testing, but a self-pay person can anticipate paying around $100 for the test. (3) The test may not be completely accurate. The titer was initially developed to quantify the serum antibodies of people with natural exposure. Natural exposure would produce all measles symptoms, and the immune system would respond accordingly. (4) Titer results are less sensitive when someone has received the immunization, often resulting in equivocal or subpar readings. These four considerations are the primary reasons why health-care providers recommend getting a booster or a third dose of MMR instead of relying on a titer.

MMR BOOSTER

Some experts recommend that individuals in high-risk groups get a booster, while others suggest that all adults receive a booster shot. The third group of experts does not recommend a booster if the person has documented proof of receiving the two-dose MMR vaccination. Dr. Nancy Messonnier, the director of the CDC's National Center for Immunization and Respiratory Diseases, stated in the article "Federal Health Officials Urge Some Adults to Get Revaccinated against Measles amid Worst Outbreak in 25 Years" (2019) that most adults are protected against measles, but that does not mean that all are. An adult in New York City recently had a titer drawn before traveling to a country with an active outbreak. The adult had documentation of the vaccination, and yet her antibody test was negative for immunity.

One factor considered relevant to the problem is the vaccine administered between 1963 and 1967 with a killed version of the virus. This vaccine was later discovered to be unable to provide lifelong immunity. Many baby boomers (born between 1946 and 1964) are unaware of the situation and vulnerable to acquiring the infection. Other experts believe that as humans age, their immune system becomes less efficient. Thus, an MMR booster would benefit the elderly (over 65) living in assisted living facilities and nursing homes. Few studies support this practice or indicate outbreaks in the United States for this populous. Although no adverse reactions have been documented from the booster, many providers believe it is not necessary. Other providers encourage the administration of an MMR booster for anyone traveling in areas with a current outbreak. Most physicians agree that high-risk groups should consider getting revaccinated, including health-care workers, those living in areas with a current outbreak, international travelers, and immunocompromised individuals.

FACTORS THAT CAN INFLUENCE THE EFFECTIVENESS OF THE IMMUNE SYSTEM

Although the MMR vaccine is considered safe and effective, some factors may negatively impact the body's ability to mount a strong immunological response to the vaccine. These factors may also impact the body's ability to combat naturally acquired measles.

Refined Sugar

The Mayo Clinic (2020) issued a statement that excessive sugar intake can reduce the body's immune defenses by 75 percent. Most people are aware that sugar has negative consequences to health, but how it impacts the immune system is less well known. The impact of consuming sugar is that the functions of the immune system decrease for two to five hours. Loma Linda University researchers investigated how the white blood cells (the cells that fight infection) are affected by sugar with astonishing results. The functions of the white blood cells decreased by approximately 50 percent after eating any form of sugar. Sugars from candy, cookies, and cakes had the same effect as processed bagels, crackers, or popcorn. All processed carbohydrates break down into sugars and cause the same detrimental issues. The consumption of one cup of cooked plain spaghetti (containing forty-three grams of carbohydrates) equals eleven teaspoons of sugar. A healthier alternative would be a cup of zucchini noodles, which has less than one teaspoon of sugar in a serving. In the book *Food: What the Heck Should I Eat?*, Dr. Mark Hyman (2018) reports that U.S. government surveys reveal that the average American consumes 152 pounds of sugar annually. This amount of sugar has a detrimental impact on the immune system.

Stress

Stress is an integral component of modern everyday life as people drive to and from work in traffic, study for a test, or care for a loved one who is ill or disabled. Stress can be both detrimental and instrumental. The positive effects of stress motivate humans to accomplish complex tasks over the short term, but it can take a toll on the immune system when such stress becomes chronic. Dr. Leonard Calabrese, a doctor of osteopathy at the Cleveland Clinic, believes that eliminating or modifying stress in one's life can protect a person from illness and aging. Dr. Calabrese has several YouTube videos and has written more than 350 peer-reviewed articles. The physician supports the belief that when a person's stress overwhelms coping skills, the body releases the hormone cortisol. A brief period of elevated cortisol boosts the immune response to inflammation. However, the body loses this benefit over the long term, and inflammation increases over time.

High-stress levels increase the risk of depression and anxiety, resulting in more inflammation, which at some point overwhelms the immune system and causes it to lose its protective qualities. The reduction of stress is known to improve the work of the immune system. The first step is to identify and mitigate known stress factors. The good news is that stress prevention can be as simple as taking a deep breath. Belly breathing is an effective method of reducing the negative qualities of stress, plus it is non-pharmacological and free. Simply sit or stand in a comfortable position. Place the hands on the abdomen and take a deep breath through the nose. Hold the breath for four seconds, then exhale with pursed lips. Then, take another deep breath. Repeat this cycle three to five times until you feel the stress dissipate. Other solutions to stress reduction include dietary changes, exercise, adequate sleep, and meditation.

OTHER FORMS OF PREVENTION

According to the CDC and the WHO, vaccines are the sole method for preventing measles. This precedence is statistically supported by the decrease of measles cases when an effective vaccination campaign exists. Despite this evidence, some people will not accept vaccination. Many do not get vaccinations for religious and philosophical beliefs. Others physically cannot receive a vaccination due to a medical condition. What alternative choices do these people have to prevent this highly contagious infection?

Science has proven that the most effective method of measles prevention is the two-dose MMR vaccine, which provides a 97 percent lifetime protection with minimal complications, so most health-care providers would say that the best prevention is vaccination. The first dose of the MMR is usually administered around one year of age and the second dose by age six. The two-dose vaccination would be the end of the story if everyone uniformly supported and adhered to this program. However, many people have not only questioned this practice but also directly opposed it.

Western medicine treats diseases and symptoms with drugs, radiation, and surgery. The book *The Social Transformation of American Medicine: The Rise of a Sovereign Profession and the Making of a Vast Industry*, by Paul Starr (1982), describes how Western medicine transitions from private practices to the hospital setting. During this time, practitioners focused on chemical solutions (pills) to control diseases. This approach continues today. However, this is not the only approach to medicine. Eastern medical practices have existed for thousands of years and are still used today. The basis of Eastern medicine is that the body's energy must be balanced to integrate the mind, body, and spirit. This holistic approach considers the conjoined elements of a living being to utilize diet, herbal therapy, massage, and meditation. Many experts in the West incorporate some of these practices and support alternative methods to vaccinations due to the current and ongoing autoimmune diseases linked to the rising number of vaccines administered.

The development of an illness-prevention strategy for the population vulnerable to measles is recommended by the WHO in several reports that highlight health promotion and primary prevention. *Health promotion* is the ability of the general public to control health and seek opportunities for improvement, and it encourages people to thoughtfully make choices in their everyday life that will enhance their overall health. Primary preventions are, according to the CDC, actions that would prevent a disability or disease. The foundation of an illness-prevention strategy must incorporate health promotion and primary prevention.

The application of three specific strategies supports the prevention of measles and improves overall health. The techniques include eating a nutrient-dense diet, providing support of the microbial cell in the digestive system, and stress reduction. Good nutrition is the foundation for overall health. The immune system relies on nutrients for cell activation and processes. Vitamins and minerals such as A, C, D, and K, along with calcium and magnesium, are of particular importance to this effort.

Many physicians in the early 1920s and 1930s believed that measles resulted from a deficiency in vitamin A. Today, the CDC and the WHO support vitamin A supplements for those diagnosed with measles, especially in developing countries. The WHO recommends administering an oral dose of 200,000 international units (IU) of vitamin A to adults and 100,000 IU to children for two consecutive days as soon as they have been diagnosed with measles—a practice that developing countries could afford. Vitamin A costs less than ten cents per dose and could prevent thousands of dollars spent on hospitalization.

A literature review was conducted in 2005 by Drs. Hui Yang, Meng Mao, and Chaomin Wan. The researchers discovered a reduced mortality rate among children less than five years of age and infected with measles who had received two doses of vitamin A. Vitamin A was also associated with a reduced risk of pneumonia and diarrhea, specifically among children less than two years of age. Subsequent studies have supported this outcome. A 2010 study published in the *International Journal of Epidemiology* by Sudfeld, Navar, and Halsey suggests that oral doses of vitamin A should be used in conjunction with the MMR vaccine.

Even more important is the vitamin A research conducted by Dr. Alfred Sommer in the 1970s. The study's original focus was on blindness in children who had a vitamin A deficiency. The investigation determined that children with a vitamin A deficiency were more ill with measles than those who did not have this deficit. Large clinical trials in 1980 and into 1990 cemented this observation and hypothesized that the inclusion of vitamin A into the diet would reduce deaths from infectious diseases. This study was the catalyst for the WHO recommending that an aggressive daily dose of vitamin A be added to the diets of children with measles.

The microbial cells in the human digestive system, also referred to as "the gut," are responsible for 80 percent of the immune systems' functionality. These cells provide a unique opportunity to recognize foreign particles and initiate a "seek and destroy mission." Chapter 5 explains the characteristics of the immune system in detail. Microbiome cells are beneficial fungi, yeast, and bacteria that usually reside in the digestive tract and assist the immune system. The saying is true, "You are unhealthy if your gut is unhealthy." The way to ensure a healthy gut is through proper nutrition, including the vitamins and minerals previously discussed. However, a healthy gut needs nutritionally dense foods that support the microbial environment, including cod liver oil, raw sauerkraut, bone broth, almonds, yogurt, green leafy vegetables, and mushrooms.

Other ways to support the microbiome are through nonfood practices, either preventing measles or reducing the infection's impact. Health-care organizations and physicians highly recommend probiotics to improve the gut environment for good bacteria and yeast. The main job of probiotics is to maintain homeostasis in the digestive tract and support the immune system. This feat is accomplished by adding in the digestion of food and the use of vitamins from foods. Probiotics also help break down and absorb medications in the digestive tract. The most important function is maintaining the epithelial cell lining and preventing harmful bacteria from entering the bloodstream. Bacteria allowed to enter the bloodstream can result in cellular damage and widespread infection.

Common probiotics such as *Lactobacillus* and *Bifidobacterium* are readily available for in-store or online purchase. *Saccharomyces boulardii* is the most common form of yeast found in probiotics. A substantial amount of research has supported probiotics, but researchers still cannot address how probiotics help many conditions. What can be reported is that people who consistently take a probiotic report few gastrointestinal complications or signs of illnesses. Conditions that specifically include diarrhea, constipation, irritable bowel syndrome, eczema, upper respiratory infections, and urinary tract infections have diminished through the application of probiotics. It is important to note that probiotics are not a medication and do not receive approval from the FDA. The manufacture of probiotics can range from drug-quality sterile environments to home (or garage) production with minimal standards. Quality probiotics are considered safe to consume. People who have a weakened immune system, who have had a recent surgery, or who are critically ill should consult with a physician before taking either probiotics or over-the-counter supplements.

Primary Prevention

The final method of prevention most important for averting measles is appropriate hygiene, such as handwashing. Consistent and effective handwashing is a vital component of any illness-prevention strategy. According to Dr. Layla McCay, the secretariat director of the Global Public-Private Partnership for Handwashing, handwashing is a particularly effective prevention that is second only to vaccination. Handwashing removes the tiny particulates that contain measles virus from the hands before transmitting the virus to the self or another through surfaces.

The CDC has identified five steps for effective handwashing. First, wet hands with running water and apply soap containing natural antibacterial products such as orange and lavender oils. The soap should be natural or organic and not include Triclosan, which is harmful to the immune system and alters hormones. Second, lather the hands, including the backs of the hands, between fingers, and under the nails. Third, scrub the hands vigorously together for twenty seconds. Twenty seconds is the length of time it takes to sing "Happy Birthday" twice. Fourth, thoroughly rinse the hands under running water. And fifth, dry the hands and turn off the water with a clean paper towel. If soap and water are unavailable, use a 60 percent alcohol-based hand sanitizer. However, sanitizers are not as effective and may not remove all germs.

In summary, measles can be safely prevented with the two-dose MMR vaccine. Still, if the vaccine is not an option due to a medical condition, personal convictions, or religious beliefs, an illness-prevention strategy is an alternative solution. The plan should include nutrient-dense foods and supplemental vitamins and minerals, especially vitamin A. The consumption of sugar should be carefully monitored, allowing the immune system to function at its optimal best. Stress reduction lowers the level of cortisol and inflammation, improving the functions of the immune system. The most crucial step in preventing virus-induced illness is handwashing, which, if done regularly and efficiently, removes the droplets containing the measles virus. Prevention is a multifaceted solution that has a synergistic effect on a person's overall health.

9

Issues and Controversies

Measles continues to be an issue in today's modern society, especially in undeveloped countries. The Measles and Rubella Initiative (MRI) is a global collaboration with preeminent health-care organizations, including the American Red Cross, the Centers for Disease Control and Prevention (CDC), the World Health Organization (WHO), and the United Nations Children's Fund (UNICEF). This collaboration reported that significant progress has been achieved, but approximately 143,000 children still die each year, most of whom are under the age of five. The question is, why are there still children dying when a scientifically proven two-dose vaccination is available that is safe and effective? The answer is both simple and complex. This simple response is that many countries do not have the infrastructure to support a successful vaccine campaign. The complex response is that many members of the general public do not believe in the science behind the vaccines and do not support vaccination.

This chapter explores some of the issues and controversies surrounding measles, mumps, and rubella (MMR) vaccination, beginning with issues concerning pregnancy and the unborn child. Allergies to the content of the MMR are defined and supported by evidence-based research. The major controversy surrounding MMR vaccines is also discussed: the presumed link between the vaccine and autism. The chapter concludes with how the issues and disputes affect measles cases on a global basis.

PREGNANT WOMEN

The immune system of a pregnant woman is in constant flux. Current research supports the theory that the immune system is an active part of pregnancy's fetal cell implementation phase. Immune cells invade the lining of the uterus and initiate the inflammatory cascade, which is a complicated response by the body to current or perceived injuries. Cells release chemicals at the site of injury, which recruit other cells to assist in the healing process. However, recruited cells resist rejection of the fetus and facilitate implantation in the uterus.

Dr. Gil Mor (2020), a professor of obstetrics, gynecology, and reproductive diseases at Yale School of Medicine, theorizes that viruses diminish or eradicate both the pregnant mother's and the unborn fetus's ability to fight infections. The virus detection signaling process can become overwhelmed and unable to interact with the virus as it usually would due to the pregnant women's immune system being activated during the pregnancy's implementation phase. Coined the "double-hit hypothesis," this theory leaves the mother and fetus at risk for preterm delivery. More than 40 percent of all preterm deliveries result from some form of infection. Even if the fetus does not succumb to the mother's disease, the highly active inflammatory marker can result in fetal abnormalities and preterm delivery. Dr. Mor suggests that research links viral infections during pregnancy with allergies, mental health disorders, and autism spectrum disorders.

Women who are planning to become pregnant should discuss their immune status with their physician, according to the American College of Obstetricians and Gynecologists (ACOG). Most physicians encourage a measles titer to quantify the current immunological position if the woman is unaware of her immune status. The ACOG recommends that unvaccinated women receive the MMR vaccine and wait four weeks before attempting pregnancy. This precaution is advised because the MMR vaccine contains a live-attenuated virus, so there is a potential (though relatively small) risk to the fetus. One dose of the MMR vaccine is sufficient for women with low-risk pregnancies. Women in geographical areas with current outbreaks and immunocompromised women should consider receiving two doses of the MMR vaccine before pregnancy. The two-dose vaccine needs a thirty-day window between inoculations with an additional thirty-day waiting period prior to conception. A consultation with an obstetrician and the local health department is warranted in these circumstances.

There is an option to reduce the viral effects to the fetus if an unvaccinated pregnant woman is exposed during pregnancy. Postexposure prophylaxis treatment with an intravenously administered immunoglobulin (IGIV) within six days of exposure can modify the virus's clinical course for the unvaccinated pregnant woman. The exact dosage is specific to each pregnant woman's weight; the usual dose for IGIV is 100–400 mg/kg for women with a low-risk pregnancy. High-risk pregnancies require additional dosage. An intravenously administered immunoglobulin injection consists of plasma pooled from a large number of healthy individuals that contains comparable levels of antigen-specific antibodies. These antibodies reduce or eliminate the viral load for the pregnant woman and the risk of the fetus's rejection (premature birth). Some obstetricians and public health agencies additionally recommend receiving the MMR vaccine within seventy-two hours of exposure. However, this practice is considered controversial by many health-care providers.

Pregnant women who contract measles from the rubella virus are at higher risk for premature labor, low birth weight, and even maternal death. Congenital rubella is spread in the bloodstream from the pregnant woman to the unborn child and is the most severe complication resulting from this condition. Congenital rubella can cause many congenital disabilities, and contracting rubella during the first trimester increases this risk. The most common congenital disabilities are cataracts, heart defects, hearing loss, and learning disabilities. The rubella virus may furthermore increase the risk of a miscarriage or stillbirth.

The first trimester of pregnancy is the most susceptible time for damage from measles. Pregnant women will have the same symptoms as the general public if they contract the virus. Measles has not been linked to congenital disabilities but can result in miscarriage, premature labor, or low birth weight. A study conducted in 2013 by the CDC explored the effects of measles with fifty-eight pregnant women and found that pregnant women have an increased risk for life-threatening complications, especially pneumonia. Of the fifty-eight women in the measles study, fifteen developed pneumonia, and two died. Thirteen of the fifty-eight pregnancies resulted in premature delivery, and five pregnancies terminated from spontaneous abortion. These risks for the fetus and the pregnant women continue throughout the entire pregnancy.

ALLERGIES TO GELATIN OR NEOMYCIN

There is minimal risk of an allergic reaction with the MMR vaccine. The World Allergy Organization explains that the MMR vaccine is grown in a culture made from chicken embryo fibroblasts. These cultures contain minimal to no egg proteins and are safe to administer to anyone, even those with egg allergies, with no special precautions. However, the rubber used to create the vaccine's vial stoppers and the plungers for the syringes that deliver the vaccine could potentially trigger an allergic reaction. Most rubber used for these two products is dry natural rubber or synthetic rubber. A small hypothetical risk exists if the recipient has a latex allergy. Anyone with a known latex allergy is still protected if the MMR vaccine was produced or marketed in the United States, as U.S. producers do not use latex. In countries that produce vaccines with latex or for women who have had a hypersensitive reaction to latex, the woman can receive treatment for the allergy before inoculation.

Many people are allergic to the gelatin in the MMR vaccine, which is used as a stabilizer. The allergic reaction in its most severe form is known as anaphylactic shock and can be life-threatening. Patients with an allergic reaction to gelatin should be referred to an allergist for further testing before administering any vaccine containing gelatin as a stabilizer. Commercially prepared assays can be used by the allergist to test the patient's allergic reactions. A crude mixture of normal saline and sugared gelatin powder (e.g., Jell-O) can serve as an assay, although the Food and Drug Administration (FDA) does not provide approval of this technique. The allergist would test the response with a skin test by scratching or pricking the skin with the gelatin test solution. A patient who tests positive for an allergy to gelatin could still receive the vaccine using a graded dose protocol of diluting the average dose volume with normal saline.

Encephalitis (swelling of the brain) has resulted in rare instances of administering the vaccine. Encephalitis begins with a fever and headache and progresses to seizures, confusion, and muscle weakness. The patient could also develop pneumonia (lung infection) or thrombocytopenia, which reduces the platelet count and causes excessive bruising and bleeding. According to the CDC, people with severe immune disorders, such as HIV, should not be vaccinated because the vaccine is a live-attenuated (weakened) virus, which could predispose the person to a severe reaction.

RECENT MEASLES OUTBREAKS

The World Health Organization (WHO) indicates that more measles cases worldwide occurred in 2019 than any year since 2006; some regions reported alarming increases. Africa had a whopping 900 percent increase, the Western Pacific region had a 230 percent increase, and Europe reported a 150 percent increase. In 2018 alone, 140,000 deaths occurred, even though the global MMR vaccination initiative resulted in a 73 percent decrease in measles deaths between 2000 and 2018. Europe reported 83,540 confirmed cases, with 74 deaths, in 2018. Ten countries have recognized a measles endemic: Belgium, Bosnia, France, Georgia, Germany, Italy, Romania, Russia, Serbia, and Ukraine. Ukraine alone had 53,218 confirmed cases just in 2018. Most of the deaths associated with measles were children under the age of five.

Outbreaks in the United States

Chapter 2 described the history of measles arriving in the Americas with Christopher Columbus, and it continued to course its destructive path until 1963, when the MMR vaccination offered hope of controlling this highly contagious disease. Measles was declared an eradicated illness in the United States after a successful vaccination crusade by the WHO in 2000. Only eighty-six measles cases were confirmed during that year. The trend did not continue, as the disease returned with a vengeance. Fifteen states reported the highest number of measles cases since 1996 eight years later, in the first six months of 2008. The battle was taking a turn for the worse.

The measles revival in the United States is associated with increased international travel to and from other countries where measles remains endemic and vaccination coverage is less available. The number of internationally imported measles cases is alarming. Internationally imported measles means that the contagious period increases from seven to twenty-one days before the onset of a rash and exposure occurred before entering the United States. Imported virus cases also have an epidemiologic link, a specific genotype associated with a geographical location or populous infection in a foreign country. By May 2011, imported measles was found in twenty-three states, with New York City having the highest occurrence. A total of eleven outbreaks were documented, with 40 percent of the cases requiring hospitalization. One of Minnesota's epidemics was noteworthy because of the twenty-one people exposed; most were children whose parents opted not to vaccinate for personal reasons. Seven infants who were too young to be vaccinated were also part of this outbreak.

Unvaccinated American travelers continued to spread measles and create local outbreaks over the next few years. Multiple states reported ongoing outbreaks, with New York State and New York City accounting for most cases. An unvaccinated adolescent traveled to London, England, while being contagious with measles in March 2013. This adolescent, considered "patient zero," was viewed as the cause of the most devastating measles outbreak since 1996. Epidemiologists identified the measles genotype using medical records, interviews, immunization records, and serum (blood) tests. This genotype matched the unvaccinated adolescent. The analysis allowed epidemiologists to link the single infected adolescent's strain of measles to fifty-eight cases.

The first person diagnosed with measles from this outbreak was identified in Brooklyn's Borough Park neighborhood of Williamsburg, which is inhabited by Orthodox Jews, all of whom had been unvaccinated. Three extended families from this community reported the early measles symptoms at the median age of ten. The outbreak spilled into Williamsburg's surrounding neighborhood, where the infection targeted children, most of whom were less than two years old. All cases had serum testing for the measles genotype and were linked to patient zero, who was a seventeen-year-old adolescent. Over 3,500 contacts were identified by the New York City Department of Health and Mental Hygiene and required notification through letters, public service announcements, and flyers.

In 2015, 127 cases of significant importance were linked to Disneyland. This outbreak highlighted the vaccination controversy. Researchers developed a mathematical model using data from the California Department of Public Health and medical records to analyze the vaccination rates among the people associated with this incident. The lead researcher, Maimuna Majumder (2015), a research fellow at Boston Children's Hospital, said this study used rigorous scientific evidence to confirm that low vaccine rates might have been the leading cause of this outbreak. The study reveals that the vaccination rate for the exposed people was as little as 50 percent. Scientists and epidemiologists have speculated that low vaccination rates have been a predisposing factor with previous outbreaks. The mathematical model has shown the potential to assist in identifying the possible cause of future episodes.

The controversy of vaccination has continued into 2018, which saw 370 confirmed measles cases scientifically connected to imported measles via genotyping in areas with reduced vaccination rates. This trend continued in 2019 with almost 900 patients, mostly in Washington and New York. The following year, 2020, began with a significant issue for the United States: according to the CDC, if the measles trend continues, there is the potential of the United States losing its measles eradication status. This loss is particularly alarming because the United States is esteemed as a global leader in public health.

Pacific Islands

The Pacific Islands have recently experienced a resurgence in measles. As of December 2019, 440 cases of confirmed or suspected measles had been reported on the small island of Tonga. The majority of these cases were boys and men between the ages of ten and twenty-four; fortunately, no deaths were reported. The island of Fiji reported fifteen confirmed measles cases, and other Pacific Islands followed the same resurgent pattern. Measles overwhelmed the health-care system in Samoa, where 4,900 people of the island's total population (200,000) were diagnosed with measles. Seventy-one died, with most of the fatalities being children under five years of age.

The WHO attributes the recent measles epidemic to a rise in tourist travel to the islands, the local population traveling between the islands, and anti-vaccine activists. The activists are responding to the deaths of two children who died shortly after receiving their first dose of the MMR vaccine in 2018, which caused the entire country to cease all vaccinations. The nurses who administered the MMR vaccine diluted the drug with a muscle relaxant instead of sterile water. Both nurses were convicted of manslaughter and are now in prison.

This situation has ramped up the anti-vaccine campaigns. The government has teamed up with Hawaii's lieutenant governor, Josh Green, to reestablish a successful vaccination crusade. The number of children with measles has overwhelmed pediatric units; many children have developed severe pneumonia as a measles complication and require mechanical ventilation. The Samoan government and public health officials are requesting additional ventilators and medical staff during this crisis. Only one-third of the children in Samoa are vaccinated.

The WHO has recommended that all the Pacific Islands develop active screening by investigating every person with a fever and a rash who seeks medical care. This process assists in ensuring an efficient and timely diagnosis. The recommendations of the WHO also urge public health officials to pledge that an effective leadership structure be developed that would allow for a rapid response to confirmed measles cases. The WHO strongly encourages the dissemination of measles cases to all public health officials and health-care facilities. A prompt response to all confirmed cases with vaccination teams would result in a swift vaccination campaign. The island must maintain adequate medical supplies to triage and treat patients diagnosed with measles, focusing on infection control and prevention. The WHO endorses a collaborative plan to reduce further measles outbreaks and pledges to institute immunization guidelines for the current population (especially children), travelers entering the islands, and health-care workers.

European Countries

The past few years have seen a surge of measles in Europe. The European Centre for Disease Prevention and Control (ECDC) said that measles could have been eliminated in 2000 if the population had adhered to the proposed immunization programs, but suboptimal vaccination coverage persisted in almost all European countries. The ECDC cites three main factors for this. The first factor is that many children and teenagers born after 1999 were not vaccinated, representing a large and vulnerable population pool of approximately four million. Few countries achieved the targeted two-dose vaccination rate of 95 percent that had been established by the WHO's vaccination initiative, further increasing the exposed population. The chance of eradicating the infection using herd immunity, as described in chapter 2, is improved by having 95 percent of the population vaccinated.

The second factor in suboptimal vaccination coverage is the progressive rate of measles among infants, children, and adults in all fourteen European countries. The median age of diagnosis has increased over the past ten years, from ten to seventeen years of age. Young adults (nineteen to twenty-one years of age) account for 39 percent of measles cases from 2016 to 2019. Infants diagnosed with measles have dramatically increased forty-four times higher than any other age group and also have the highest death rate from measles at approximately 45 percent.

The third and last factor to affect measles in Europe is the enormous potential of cross contamination with bordering countries. Traveling from countries with a current measles outbreak to an uninfected area can cause an epidemic or exacerbate an existing episode. Approximately 43 percent of Europe's cases were from another European country where measles was currently having an endemic between 2016 and 2019. This cyclic effect can only be thwarted through isolation or vaccination.

From 2016 to 2019, 44,074 measles cases were confirmed in Europe, indicating that Europe needs to achieve the target of 95 percent coverage with the two-dose MMR vaccine to provide herd immunity for those who cannot be vaccinated, according to Vytenis Andriukaitis, the European commissioner for Health and Food Safety. He advocates that all children get vaccinated based on the scheduled guidelines by the WHO. Maintenance of vaccination status for intercountry travels could reduce or eliminate the outbreaks in Europe.

A lack of confidence in vaccine safety is reportedly the most common reason for the current measles resurgence based on the Vaccine Confidence Project (VCP), a global organization. The VCP surveyed 300,000 individuals using the Vaccine Confidence Index survey. France was hit the hardest of all the European countries battling the measles epidemic. Most of their 2,500 cases in 2018 were unvaccinated children. Forty-one of the French participants did not believe that vaccines were safe, according to the VCP. This belief was echoed by Italy, which had more than 3,000 cases, and Greece, with 3.039. All three countries, France, Italy, and Greece, are plagued with a low vaccination rate and are currently suffering measles epidemics. The Baltic and Scandinavian countries, by contrast, have mandated vaccination and reported only a few measles cases.

South Africa

Measles was considered eradicated from South Africa after the intense vaccination program that began in 1975. A vaccination campaign in 1996 to 1997 targeted all children between nine months and fourteen years, using the Pan American Health Organization's (PAHO) strategies. The campaign achieved its goal of an 85 percent administration rate. They met another lofty goal in 2002 of vaccinating 92 percent of children from nine months to four years old. The results of measles surveillance from 1999 to 2002 revealed less than sixty confirmed cases with no deaths. A surge of measles cases was reported from 2003 to 2007 and linked to South Africa's rising human immunodeficiency virus (HIV) status. The high HIV prevalence reduced the MMR vaccine's efficacy, and measles once again became endemic in the country.

A measles epidemic occurred in three South African provinces in 2003 that lasted for more than two years, totaling 3,000 cases and forty-six deaths. Most victims were less than five years of age. The government issued a directive to provide a booster vaccination for all children from six months to fourteen years of age. The order successfully vaccinated 85 percent of children under the age of fourteen and substantially decreased transmission rates. A collaborative study conducted by the WHO, the CDC, epidemiologists, and pediatricians showed the importance of herd immunity to protect immunocompromised children, specifically those diagnosed with HIV. The conclusion suggested that vaccination programs are highly effective but that a measles diagnosis should be augmented with vitamin D and isolation.

Other Measles Outbreaks

Measles continues to propagate on a global basis. Death rates dropped an average of 75 percent from 2000 and 2013 through vaccination campaigns by the WHO and individual countries. However, the WHO reports that measles is still a leading global cause of death for young children, specifically those under age five.

A relatively new controversy was described in a study by Italian scientists Filippo Trentini and Piero Poletti and colleagues (2019). The scientists predicted a 50 percent rise of measles by 2050 due to the phenomena known as the *elimination threshold.* The measles elimination threshold is based on the minimum percentage of immune people in the general population, which is 93–95 percent of the people. The group must have natural immunity or have received the two-dose MMR vaccine. The scientists input the current measles immunity profile and immunization strategies and statistically proposed a model for 2018 to 2050 using a quantitative research approach. The results indicated that only Singapore and South Korea would remain in the 93–95 percent range. A compulsory vaccination strategy was the only suggestion that could reduce or eradicate measles for the United Kingdom, Ireland, the United States, and Australia.

Some high-income countries, including Singapore and South Korea, have already established herd immunity and still report measles outbreaks. Dr. Poletti suggests that mandatory vaccination for all elementary school-aged children is desired for high-income countries with effective vaccination programs. Dr. Adam Finn at the University of Bristol, by contrast, proposes that mandatory vaccination at any age may not improve coverage (Science Media Centre, 2019). Some countries do not struggle with having access to vaccines; they battle with vaccine hesitancy and misconceptions. The controversies surrounding vaccination can only be addressed after providing full disclosure to the public on all MMR vaccine benefits and side effects.

There are numerous barriers to controlling measles throughout the world. It is apparent that current elimination goals are either inadequate or need to be redefined. In many countries, compulsory vaccination has produced positive effects by raising the proportion of children's immune status, but it cannot be the only strategy. Even in countries where the WHO indicates that herd immunity has been achieved, outbreaks disproportionately continue. Studies suggest that a review of the vaccination schedule may be needed, which is discussed in detail in chapter 10. Revision of the vaccination schedule coupled with a global education initiative may increase vaccination compliance.

VACCINATION AND AUTISM

Autism spectrum disorder (ASD), or autism, is a developmental disorder that disrupts behavior and communication. The exact cause of ASD is unknown, but substantial research supports a significant genetic component. A person with ASD will communicate, learn, and behave differently than someone without ASD; their abilities can range from severely challenged to gifted. ASD is an umbrella term that includes Asperger's syndrome, pervasive developmental disorder, and autistic disorder. Autism is the disorder most commonly associated with the MMR vaccine.

The autistic child exhibits a noticeable lack of eye contact and abnormal responses to stimuli, such as toys and siblings. The child may be delayed with verbal skills or have repetitive speech (perseveration). Changes in their routine, unusual sounds, and environmental stimuli elicit exaggerated responses from the autistic child. Abnormal and repetitive body movements (stimming) are frequent and include spinning, rocking, or hand flapping (asterixis).

Infants and young children with typical development patterns are curious about their world and seek interaction with touch and copying gestures, but the autistic child has a withdrawn personality, minimal to no desire for physical interaction, and a flat affect (no expression). Approximately 80–90 percent of parents with autistic children report healthy physical and intellectual development until the child's first birthday, whereupon gradual and subtle changes occur. By the age of two, many autistic children stop learning new skills or lose previously acquired skills.

Controversy has surrounded the potential link between autism and childhood vaccinations over the past two centuries and continues today. The impetus for the discussion in recent times originated with a study published in 1998 in the British medical journal *The Lancet*. The lead researcher for the study was Andrew Wakefield, a former British gastroenterologist who attended King Edward's School of Bath and graduated from Saint Mary's Hospital Medical School (now the Imperial College School of Medicine) in 1981. He subsequently became a fellow of the Royal College of Surgeons until 1985. He began his career studying small intestinal transplantation using animal models and then worked with the Royal Free Hospital's liver transplant program in London. Dr. Wakefield achieved notoriety in 1993 with a report indicating the measles vaccine might cause Crohn's disease. This study was deemed inconclusive after a group of British experts failed to support his hypothesis in 1998, though the research became known in the medical community. A mother named Rosemary Kessick sought assistance from Dr. Wakefield in 1996 for her son, who had bowel problems and autism (Frankel, 2004). Ms. Kessick had established a support group called Allergy Induced Autism and was supporting a link between gastrointestinal issues, autism, and environmental triggers. Dr. Wakefield began looking for a connection between autism and the MMR vaccine based on this meeting.

This connection was the impetus for a study conducted in 1998 at the Royal Free Hospital and School of Medicine on twelve children with chronic enterocolitis and regressive development disorder, including communication. Dr. Wakefield was the lead researcher for a team of thirteen scientists. The parents of eight of the participants attributed their children's symptoms to the MMR vaccine injection. Based on the parents' beliefs, the researchers concluded their study by stating that "possible environmental triggers" (the MMR vaccine) caused a gastrointestinal disorder termed as "autistic enterocolitis" and developmental regression known as "autism." Interestingly, the children of this study were between one to two years of age, which is the recommended time for the first MMR vaccine, explaining the association between autism and the injection.

It was determined that this research had been conducted under questionable circumstances. The participants for the research had been carefully selected, not randomly selected, and the children's parents were also part of a lawsuit against the vaccine's manufacturers. Some of Dr. Wakefield's research funding came from the lawyers involved in this lawsuit. Dr. Wakefield made controversial statements at a press conference on the research results, concluding that the MMR vaccine should be suspended until additional research was done. An article by Andy Coghlan (2010) reported that Dr. Wakefield said it was a "moral issue" and that "if you give three viruses together, three live viruses, then you potentially increase the risk of an adverse event occurring, particularly when one of those viruses influences the immune system in the way that measles does.

A British investigative reporter, Brian Deer, presented evidence in 2004 that Dr. Wakefield had fabricated some research data, whereupon the editors of *The Lancet* issued a statement that supported the study's results and found no evidence that the researchers had been aware of the existence of ongoing litigation. Subsequent studies failed to corroborate Dr. Wakefield's results, including a 1999 British study, a 2002 research project in Denmark, and a 2005 Japanese study. A total of ten research studies were unable to reproduce the same results. Australian scientists Luke Taylor, Amy Swerdfeger, and Guy Eslick (2014) reviewed and analyzed the ten inquiries, encompassing a total of 1.2 million children, and found no relationship between vaccines and autism. The results prompted an additional investigation into the original research by Dr. Wakefield.

Twelve years after its initial publication, *The Lancet* began another investigation and discovered questionable and unethical practices. *The Lancet* officially retracted the research as having been based on contrary and incorrect findings. Ten of the studies' original authors signed a formal retraction and renounced the research conclusions. A retraction is a rare event that proclaims that the paper should not be part of scientific evidence. This particular research was found to be fraudulent and misrepresented the data collected. Britain's General Medical Council reviewed the research study and found that Dr. Wakefield and his associates had conducted the study using unethical practices and disregarded the children's safety. Dr. Wakefield was immediately suspended from practicing medicine in the United Kingdom, and his name was removed from the medical registry. The physician reported that his suspension was a result of the undesirable consequences of his research.

The withdrawal of the inquiry did little to change the opinion of many parents with autistic children. Dr. Jeanette Holden, a geneticist at the Queen's University in Canada, and Dr. Suzanne Lewis, a pediatrician and professor at the University of British Columbia in Vancouver, are both members of the Autism Spectrum Disorders Canadian-American Research

Consortium, and they supported the retraction of the study. Both physicians believe that families of autistic children are searching for a cause for autism. Autism has a genetic link, but there are additional environmental factors that have not been adequately addressed. Still, many parents remain convinced that the MMR vaccine is a causal factor.

Dr. Wakefield and his colleagues continued to suggest that there is a definitive link between autism and the MMR vaccine. The researchers used intestinal biopsies to test for measles in children with and without measles in a subsequent 2002 study. The study had ninety-one participants; sixteen of the children had tested negative for measles and not been diagnosed with autism. All the intestinal biopsies tested positive for measles among the remaining seventy-five participants. A disproportionate number of children were diagnosed with autism (70 out of the 75). Only five children had positive intestinal biopsies and tested negative for measles.

The research had the same lack of reliability and validity as Dr. Wakefield's previous study. Reliability and validity are two standards used to confirm the quality of research. *Reliability* indicates the consistency of the results of the study and measurements used for the analysis. *Validity* refers to the accuracy of the measurements and whether the inquiry is measuring what it claims to measure. England was experiencing an outbreak during the time of the study, and yet the researchers did not determine or even take into consideration whether the children with positive intestinal biopsies had natural measles or tested positive from the MMR injection. It was expected that children who had received the MMR vaccine would naturally have positive intestinal results. The antigen-presenting cells (APCs) of those who have been vaccinated travel throughout the body, including the intestinal tract, an integral part of the immune system. The study should have provided additional details, such as immunization status (natural immunity or MMR vaccine) and children with and without autism, to be considered valid and reliable. This data was omitted from the research results, even though it was available through medical records.

The study would have additionally needed to be conducted as blinded to prevent biased results. Blinded research studies do not allow the person who processed the biopsies to know information regarding the participants, thus allowing for anonymity. No mention of this was included in the inquiry. The qualification parameter for verification of the biopsy results was excluded in the final analysis. The investigation did expose an alarming statistical link between autistic children and measles, but regressive analysis of the study by other scientists has attempted to explain that these results were due to the timing of MMR vaccination and not the vaccine itself.

Several ecological studies have addressed the link between the MMR vaccine and autism. Researchers in the United Kingdom evaluated computerized health records of 498 autistic children born between 1979 and 1992. The study specifically examined the rate of an autism diagnosis after 1987, when the MMR vaccine was introduced. The scientists did not observe a change in the percentage of children with autism when the children received their MMR vaccination.

Another study conducted in the United Kingdom used the General Practice Research Database. This database is an extensive collection of medical records that includes vaccination data. Over three million people were observed from 1988 to 1999 for a spike in autistic diagnosis due to the MMR vaccination campaign that began in 1987. The analysis did not indicate an increase in autism. Duplication of this study in California (1980–1994) used the California Department of Developmental Services database. The inquiry results validated the United Kingdom's research; the increase in autism did not correlate with measles immunization. Canadian researchers conducted a similar study on close to 30,000 children in Quebec. The results surprisingly indicated a decrease in autism when there was an increase in the MMR vaccination rate.

Four retrospective observational studies explored the connection between the MMR vaccine and autism. Researchers in the United Kingdom could not identify a difference between visits to their primary practitioner for cognitive concerns with the control group (71 MMR-vaccinated children) and the case group (248 MMR-vaccinated children). Researchers examined close to 540 vaccination records and could not link an autistic disorder diagnosis with the timing of the MMR vaccination. Scientists in Denmark observed the relationship between the date of the MMR inoculation and the development of autistic symptoms in close to the same number of children born from 1991 to 1998. Their study did not produce a connection between autism and the time of vaccination.

ANTI-VACCINATION MOVEMENTS

The question remains, why do parents choose not to vaccinate their children with an inexpensive and safe vaccine? The investigation into the issue reveals that the answer is both simple and complex. The simple response is that some parents do not believe in vaccination for philosophical or religious reasons. The complex response is that many parents fear harming their children. Thus, the anti-vaccination movements enter the health-care picture. Some people have a general distrust of all medical professionals. Others relish conspiracy theories that involve the government, big pharmaceutical companies, or any form of organization that mandates vaccinations. There are also groups that suspect genocide for minority populations or those that are considered tainted or different than the "normal" population, like the mentally ill or intellectually impaired.

Distrust in vaccinations was warranted early on in the history of immunizations. Many of the early vaccinations were produced under questionable situations and often provided minimal protection paired with a high risk for complications. Inoculations were banned by the French Parliament due to the Italian Dr. Gatti's unsanitary inoculation practices of 1763. Three years later, Edward Jenner developed what he called a smallpox vaccine, but it turned out that he was unintentionally inoculating for cowpox. A legitimate concern that the vaccine production was unsanitary and therefore resulted in secondary infections also circulated. The clergy in the 1700s and 1800s did not support inoculations for smallpox because they believed that the disease was God's punishment and should be untreated.

The status of measles eradication in the United States is slowly slipping away because anti-vaccination movements have expanded and increased the risk of contracting measles. Many religious communities, such as the Amish in the Midwest and Orthodox Jews in New York City and New York State, have up to 90 percent of their communities unvaccinated. Most of these communities are isolated geographically with minimal interaction with those outside their religious group; nevertheless, they remain at high risk for a measles outbreak within their own communities.

Most states allow parents to opt out of vaccinating their children for philosophical or religious beliefs, but five states have revisited this policy due to recent outbreaks. New York, California, Maine, Mississippi, and West Virginia have passed laws that require children attending public schools to be vaccinated unless there is a documented medical condition that would allow an exemption. Conversely, Minnesota is very lenient and even allows parents to refuse all vaccinations for their children for personal beliefs. The number of confirmed measles cases is expected to rise exponentially relative to the rise in the number of unvaccinated children.

Other anti-vaccination groups are focused on the physical content of the vaccinations. Known as Green Our Vaccines, the organization suggests that the MMR vaccine is unsafe because it contains thimerosal as a preservative and preventative for the growth of bacteria. Concerns arise with this preservative because thimerosal contains trace amounts of mercury. The use of thimerosal was discontinued in the United States in 2001, but it is still used in the multidose flu vials and diphtheria, tetanus, and pertussis vaccine (Tdap). No studies have reported a direct link of thimerosal to autism or any significant complication, but as a precautionary measure, the U.S. Public Health Service recommended the removal of this substance from all childhood vaccines.

Another proposed conspiracy theory states that vaccine manufacturers do not disclose all the facts surrounding the vaccine. This theory has spawned several online groups to argue that all childhood vaccinations are unsafe, such as the prominent blog site of the Age of Autism. This group states on its website that excessive vaccine injections are the real cause of autism. The group admits that unvaccinated children can develop autism but emphasizes that other environmental factors, such as toxic chemicals, are also contributory.

Generation Rescue is a nonprofit organization founded in 2005 and supported by celebrities such as Jenny McCarthy and Jim Carrey. The organization supports the belief that the MMR vaccine causes autism and backs Dr. Wakefield's study from 1998. The organization also linked the preservative thimerosal, which contains mercury, with autism. Dr. Wakefield is a spokesperson for Generation Rescue and its Miracle Mineral Solution, which purportedly cures autism.

Dr. Wakefield has continued to support the belief that autism is a direct result of vaccines. This belief was recently expressed in a self-directed documentary titled *Vaxxed: From Cover-Up to Catastrophe*. The film reportedly offers a conclusive link of autism with childhood vaccinations and was set to premiere at the 2016 Tribeca Film Festival. *Vaxxed* is a documentary that claims the CDC orchestrated a conspiracy to cover up the link between autism and the MMR vaccine. Congressman Bill Posey also supports this conspiracy theory. He actively advocated for a full investigation of the CDC and the alleged fraudulent activities, especially with the MMR vaccine and autism link. *Vaxxed* was removed from the Tribeca Film Festival program for reasons not disclosed.

The anti-vaccination controversy was part of the 2016 presidential campaign. During a 2015 debate for the Republican Party, nominee-elect Donald J. Trump was asked whether he supported the vaccine. He responded that the MMR, a triple shot, could be the cause of autism. Politico quoted Trump as saying, "You take this little, beautiful baby and you pump—it's meant for a horse, not for a child." Trump added that autism has become an "epidemic" in recent decades. In response to the 2019 measles outbreak in California, President Trump told CNN's Joe Johns in an interview a different opinion, and that he is encouraging parents to get their children vaccinated.

Dr. Alan Palmer, a doctor of chiropractic medicine, is a well-known physician in sports injuries who offers a different perspective. Dr. Palmer's book *Truth Will Prevail* (2019) hypothesizes that over 1,200 research studies refute five of the key points that support vaccinations, including the MMR vaccine:

1.   Without the MMR vaccine, thousands of children will die.
2.   Lifelong protection is the result of the two-dose MMR regimen.

3. Booster shots will protect adults with suboptimal antibody protection.
4. Herd immunity is sustainable, with a 95 percent vaccination rate.
5. All strains of measles are addressed with the injection of the MMR and MMRV vaccines.

Dr. Palmer believes that point one is propaganda by the pharmaceutical industry to increase revenue. He believes that children should be exposed to measles and that vitamin A and other naturally derived antiviral compounds will shorten the infection and produce no adverse effects. Even the WHO promotes vitamin A supplements, especially in countries where measles is an epidemic. He asserts that correcting malnutrition and poor sanitation alone would decrease the spread of the contagious infection.

Dr. Palmer provides statistics refuting point two, showing that our immune system declines by approximately 10 percent each year as we age. This decline in antibody levels promotes vulnerability. A 2017 study published in the *Vaccine* journal and a 2018 article published in the *Journal of Infectious Disease* both agree that age decreases immunologic resistance and leaves a large portion of the adult population vulnerable to measles. A research study presented in the 2017 *Journal of Infectious Disease* demonstrated minimal effectiveness, leading the authors to state that such booster shots should be considered temporarily effective at only four months. Point three states that booster shots will protect adults with suboptimal measles antibodies. This statement is not thoroughly refuted. As adults age, the efficiency of the immune system decreases, and adults in high-risk geographical areas should receive a booster. There is minimal risk associated with the booster shot.

The fourth point addresses herd immunity. The concept of herd immunity is that the vaccinated population would offer passive protection for those not vaccinated. However, if Dr. Palmer's statistics on the declining immunity status and antibody levels of those over age sixty-five years are correct, then the herd immunity theory is moot. Cross exposure would occur between young children, fully protected adults, and those with declining or no protection.

The fifth and final point is the most perplexing. Evidence is emerging to show that measles is mutating in response to the vaccinations. An article by Munoz-Alia, Muller, and Russell (2017) in the *Journal of Virology* identified a new strain called D4.2. The D4.2 is a subgenotype mutant strain that is not responsive to the current MMR vaccine. Scientists call these strains "escape mutants," and they are currently found in France and Great Britain. The measles virus consequently seems to be surviving and morphing to continue its existence despite all efforts to eradicate it.

The anti-vaccination movement has a long history of distrust in inoculations. This distrust was warranted for some situations because vaccine manufacturing lacked evidence-based protocols for manufacturing and quality standards in the early years such that the vaccine caused more harm than good for some. Continued education of the general public about vaccines may help improve vaccine compliance by decreasing uncertainties and fears surrounding the MMR vaccine. Although many states still offer exemptions for religious or philosophical issues, there continues to be a debate between the government's need to protect society as a whole and individuals' right for self-care.

THE CONTROVERSY CONTINUES

The complications and potential disabilities of measles can have devastating effects on the social, financial, and emotional well-being of those diagnosed. People who contract measles find their immune systems weakened and experience increases in the risk of secondary complications such as pneumonia or gastrointestinal or neurological issues. Approximately 30 percent of persons with measles will have one or more long-term side effect. Disabilities are most common among children less than five years of age and unvaccinated adults over age twenty.

United States

The fact that measles is a highly contagious and debilitating virus is undeniable. It is also undeniable that this illness is preventable with a safe and inexpensive vaccine. The question is, why is the United States still plagued with this illness? Dr. Nancy Messonnier, the director of the National Center for Immunization and Respiratory Diseases at the CDC, addressed this question during a hearing with the House Energy and Commerce Subcommittee on Oversight Investigations in 2019. Dr. Messonnier responded that although some vaccination hesitancy is the result of the anti-vaccination movement, other causes are related to the U.S. healthcare system's current infrastructure, as those without health insurance find access to vaccinations limited or unavailable. Dr. Messonnier also points to hubs of community outbreaks from isolated populations of religious sects that do not support childhood vaccinations. Seventeen states currently provide parents with an opportunity to refuse vaccinations for their children for religious reasons. This statement is not to imply that religion is responsible for all of the current measles cases, but that misinformation or the lack of education may be to blame.

Dr. Anthony Fauci, the head of the National Institute of Allergy and Infectious Diseases, was in attendance at the same hearing as Dr. Messonnier. Dr.

Fauci was invited to offer his opinion on why measles is still a devastating virus in the United States. He responded that parents received insufficient or inaccurate information when making vaccine decisions and that a message based on scientific evidence was needed. Both Dr. Fauci and Dr. Messonnier concede that vaccination is a political issue that can only be resolved with an agreement between the community and government that the immunization of the majority of the general public can effectively control the number of measles cases through herd immunity, whereby those who cannot be vaccinated will have some degree of passive protection. When most of the community rejects this policy, they endanger those who are vulnerable, including infants and immunocompromised persons. Failure to accept vaccinations is a political act that affects others sharing common spaces.

Globally

The WHO has identified public mistrust as the most significant barrier to vaccinations based on the Wellcome Trust Survey. The survey was conducted in over 140 countries with greater than 140,000 responses. The survey asks whether the respondent believes that vaccines work. Eighty-four percent of the respondents indicated that they strongly or somewhat agreed with that statement. But only 79 percent of respondents thought that vaccination was safe. Even with overwhelming evidence, vaccines are the best defense against certain diseases. Vaccines have eradicated small-pox and significantly reduced the number of children diagnosed with polio. Measles was on a positive trajectory until the early 2000s. According to Dr. Ann Lindstrand, an immunization expert with WHO, vaccine hesitancy began to hinder the progress with a wide variety of vaccine-preventable diseases, including measles. The data collected by the WHO shows an increase in most regions of worldwide cases from 2016 to 2017. During these years, measles increased more than 30 percent. The rise of measles cases jeopardized the protection of the vulnerable population through herd immunity, which requires 95 percent of the population to be vaccinated.

Surprisingly, the lack of vaccine trust is from the higher-income populations such as France, where they currently have a measles outbreak and one in three residents disagreed that vaccines were safe, according to the Wellcome Trust Survey. This statistic was the highest percentage from any country participating and echoes the sentiment of most Europeans. Due to the large number of parents who do not vaccinate their children, the French government has decreed that some vaccines are not mandatory. The Italian government passed a law that unvaccinated children are banned from public schools in response to dwindling immunization rates in that country. Matt Hancock, the health secretary for the United Kingdom, is considering compulsory vaccinations if the vaccine rates continue to decline. Many Middle-European countries, such as Ukraine, Belarus, Moldova, and Russia, are experiencing a high number of measles cases. Correspondingly, vaccination compliance is below the WHO's recommendation in these countries, and approximately 50 percent of the population believes that vaccines are unsafe.

The Wellcome Trust Survey did not explore the specific reasons for low confidence in vaccines, but the researchers believe that there many. Measles has become less common in some countries, and the population has become complacent. Misinformation is easily disseminated with the widespread use of the internet, which rapidly spreads information that is often based on opinions and not scientific research. Another reason is that all medications have side effects and the fear of having an adverse reaction impedes vaccination compliance. Dr. Lindstrand believes that scientifically based education is the most effective tool to combat vaccination hesitancy, beginning with health-care workers. With knowledge, health-care workers can correctly respond to concerns that patients, parents, and the community are expressing.

10

Current Research and Future Directions

Current research on measles is being conducted to address the ongoing debate on vaccine safety. Safety in the manufacturing process and the effective administration of all vaccines were recommended by the Centers for Disease Control and Prevention (CDC) in 2014. A possible link between vaccines to cognitive disorders, such as autism, remains controversial. A vast array of research supporting and resolving the link between vaccines and autism is available for consideration, even though the scientific proof one way or the other remains inconclusive. The first year of a child's life revolves around pediatrician visits for routine wellness checkups and vaccinations if the parents decide in favor of immunizations. A child celebrating his or her first birthday will have received fifteen vaccinations following the schedule recommended by the CDC. This aggressive schedule of vaccinations has raised concerns by parents and the medical community: are there too many vaccinations being given too soon?

Biomedical research has made significant medical discoveries since the 1900s. Hundreds of lives have been saved through advanced practices such as bone marrow transplants and vaccines. Researchers in this area of expertise investigated the cause of a disease and postulated possible ways to control or eradicate the illness. One exciting outcome of this biomedical research is the development of an alternative to traditional vaccinations, including the microarray patch and inhaled vaccines. Other researchers are exploring the effectiveness of the current vaccination schedule and whether early inoculation is needed for infants. The most current and timely studies are conducted by scientists seeking a connection between the MMR vaccine and COVID-19. Exciting and promising research may hold the key to controlling one or both diseases.

The *Global Measles and Rubella Strategic Plan, 2012–2020*, was established by the World Health Organization (WHO) to eradicate measles in all nations by 2020. The organization did not meet this goal, but the vaccination campaigns derived from the effort and applied by health professionals have dramatically reduced the number of confirmed cases and measles deaths. This chapter delves into the specifics of vaccine safety and the administration schedule. It also addresses the concern that the MMR vaccine could cause autism. An understanding of current biomedical research assists future developments and new discoveries in the battle with viruses and vaccination.

VACCINE SAFETY

Vaccine safety has been a concern since the very beginning of vaccine use, but most recently, it has become the topic of numerous stories and blogs both for and against its use on the internet. Many organizations and individuals support vaccines and proclaim their safety, while others oppose the universal application on the claim they cause developmental disorders such as autism. Vaccines are held to standards that have been established by the Food and Drug Administration (FDA). The pathway for approval begins with an Investigational New Drug (IND) application. The application describes the vaccine, the manufacturing process, and the quality protocol for its release to be administered to the public. The application must also include the immunogenicity (immune response) found in animal testing and a protocol for human clinical trials.

The next step is prelicensure clinical trials with humans, which occur in three phases. Phase I begins with pilot studies using a small number of carefully monitored human subjects. Phase II involves many human subjects to assist in evaluating dosing ranges based on various parameters determined by the researchers. Phase III consists of the assembly of thousands of human participants to determine the efficacy of Phase II dosage ranges and side effects, all of which is scientifically managed to reflect the highest quality of statistical rigor. The FDA may challenge the study at any phase and require additional testing or even close the clinical trials.

A Biologics License Application (BLA) is reviewed by a multidisciplinary team of experts for validity and reliability upon satisfactory completion of all three clinical phases. The group of experts for this review includes medical practitioners, microbiologists, chemists, and FDA reviewers who debate the risks and benefits of the proposed vaccine. At the conclusion of their review, the team presents their consensual recommendation, either to approve or oppose the vaccine. If the vaccine is accepted, product labeling for health-care providers who will administer it must address usage, storage, delivery methods, and potential safety concerns. These administrators of the vaccine must clearly discuss the benefits and risks of the vaccine to each recipient.

The final step in the process of licensure is to present the findings to an independent expert committee such as the FDA's Vaccines and Related Biological Products Advisory Committee (VRBPAC). A consumer representative additionally offers a personal opinion. The FDA maintains stringent standards as it continues to oversee the medication and vaccine production in the United States. Manufacturers must submit test results confirming the potency and purity for each vaccine lot. This is a massive undertaking because all potential adverse effects cannot be determined as thousands of participants receive the vaccine during clinical trials. Phase IV requires researchers to monitor any problems found with the administration of the vaccine to the general public. This process is essential because it promotes transparency and consistency with all vaccines to promote confidence and acceptance.

Vaccine Adverse Event Reporting

The Vaccine Adverse Event Reporting System (VAERS) is a national surveillance program that oversees vaccine safety under the collaborative umbrella of the CDC and FDA. The program provides a warning system for safety issues with vaccines administered and manufactured in the United States by collecting adverse events reported by health-care providers. Anyone can report a possible health problem after receiving a vaccination, including a nurse, doctor, or parent). VAERS officials use these reports to detect "signals" indicating potential safety risks, as they systematically read each report and monitor for trends and unusual patterns in aggregate.

Anyone who receives a vaccine and subsequently has an adverse reaction or who reports this to an administrator of the vaccine is encouraged to complete a VAERS form online or by mail. Each reported event is assigned an identification number and disseminated to the reporting party. Medical records are obtained and used to evaluate each event. A follow-up letter is subsequently sent one year postevent to assess the recovery status of the patient. Injuries directly linked to vaccination may be eligible for compensation by the National Vaccine Injury Compensation Program (NVICP), which operates independently of the VAERS. The separation of the two organizations prevents any conflict of interest or biases related to the potential compensation process.

Around 3,000 VAERS reports are filed yearly, with 85–90 percent of the statements describing mild side effects, such as pain at the injection site, low-grade fever, or irritability in young children. Serious side effects include hospitalization, permanent disability, or death, which account for 10–15 percent of the VAERS reports. Each report is categorically evaluated; however, it is often difficult to determine the exact cause with many severe conditions due to patient comorbidities. The strength of VAERS lies in the centralized collection of potential vaccine safety concerns. The limitation of VAERS is the quality of the data collected and the inability to analyze the data for specific populations or geographical areas.

Vaccine Compliance Issues

Three prominent American physicians collaborated on describing issues of vaccine safety: Dr. Heather Monk Bodenstab is a clinical pharmacy specialist at the Children's Hospital of Philadelphia, Dr. Frank DeStefano is an epidemiologist and researcher for the CDC and director of the Immunization Safety Office, and Dr. Paul A. Offit is a pediatrician specializing in vaccines, infectious diseases, and virology and coinventor of the rotavirus vaccine. Together, they wrote the article titled "Principal Controversies in Vaccine Safety in the United States" (2019), which was published in the *Journal of Clinical Infectious Diseases*. These imminent providers identified seven key components that continue to affect vaccine compliance and the subsequent resurgence of vaccine-preventable infections.

The first and most damaging controversy to the MMR vaccine's safety is the supposition of a link to autism, even though a plethora of scientifically based studies have provided conclusive evidence that the MMR vaccine does not cause autism. Even so, some parents and the general public cling to the belief that there is an association between the MMR vaccine and the onset of autism—in part due to questionable practitioners who provide the "science" to support it. This unfounded belief, derived from coincidental incidence rather than direct proof, has caused parents to refuse to vaccinate their children, resulting in a resurgence in measles worldwide. Concerns about the MMR vaccine were raised in a study published in *The Lancet* in 1998. The original article was later retracted by the journal based on unethical practices with participant recruitment and financial conflict of interest. Despite a coincidental link to some children having behavioral problems after receiving the MMR vaccine, the study did not offer conclusive evidence. However, the study generated intense media coverage and public attention, despite rigorous scientific proof that the MMR vaccine does not cause autism.

Another barrier to vaccine compliance concerns the preservative thimerosal, which contains ethylmercury. Bacterial contamination of childhood vaccines was a troublesome issue in the early twentieth century. Contamination was associated with vaccines being produced in multidose vials and prepared under suboptimal hygienic conditions. A 1916 batch of typhoid vaccine was stored incorrectly, causing sixty-eight severe reactions, twenty-six abscesses, and four deaths in Columbia, South Carolina. It was apparent that an effective preservative was needed, so thimerosal entered the vaccine manufacturing process because it not only inhibited bacterial growth but also improved the efficacy of the vaccine. The concentration required for this preservative was a minuscule amount, only 1:10,000 per vial.

Thimerosal has continued to be the preservative used by vaccine manufacturers with minimal to no concerns about its safety. However, due to unsafe levels of organomercurial methylmercury found in some fish, general fears over poisoning have spilled over into all compounds containing mercury. Many anti-vaccination groups began the "Green Our Vaccines" public campaign to remove this substance, even though no studies supported the general opinion that thimerosal was harmful. Vaccine manufacturers responded to this concern by agreeing to either reduce the amount used or eliminate the material. The combination of the vaccination-autism controversy and public outcry over thimerosal was the basis for the "anti-vaxxer" movement in the United States. Jenny McCarthy, a celebrity, joined the anti-vaxxer movement when her son developed autism. She believed that her son's autism was a direct result of the MMR vaccination he had received containing the mercury-laden thimerosal preservative.

Many parents of autistic children still believe autism is caused by vaccinations, even though thimerosal was removed from vaccines in 1999. The Environmental Protection Agency (EPA) initiated a formal inquiry into cumulative mercury levels found in diphtheria-tetanus-acellular pertussis (Tdap), *Haemophilus influenzae* type b, and hepatitis B vaccines, which could cause neurological deficits in infants less than six months of age. Bacterial contamination of childhood vaccines had been a troublesome issue in the early twentieth century when contamination was associated with vaccines being produced in multidose vials and prepared under suboptimal hygienic conditions.

According to the WHO, multiple studies have not shown an increase in autism for children who received vaccinations containing thimerosal. The EPA, the American Academy of Pediatrics, and the CDC released a joint statement in 1999 to cease all vaccines containing thimerosal. A group of parents of autistic children responded by demanding extensive research on the mercury and autism correlation, which led to the eight studies on the association by the Institute of Medicine from 2001 to 2018. Two of the studies supported the theory that mercury did increase cognitive disabilities, but not specifically autism. This conclusion was a retrospective study using data before thimerosal was removed from the MMR vaccine. Even though thimerosal removal did not decrease the number of autistic diagnoses, many anti-vaxxers still claim that vaccines cause autism.

Aluminum salts are another vaccine additive that has raised concerns, as this substance is used as an adjuvant to boost the immune response. Macrophagic myofasciitis is a condition that presents with systemic complaints and generic pain. Muscle biopsies from patients suffering this condition have revealed aluminum salts found in minute lesions. Other fatigue complaints have been associated with aluminum salts, but a definitive link between aluminum and such debilitating conditions has not been established.

Guillain-Barré syndrome (GBS) has inconsistently been associated with certain vaccinations, such as the swine flu and influenza vaccines. However, there remain concerns that all vaccines increase the risk factor for this syndrome, which is a rare disorder mediated by the immune system with progressive paralysis and muscle atrophy. The symptoms begin in the feet with neurological pain and weakness, which proportionately travels up the legs. Once the disease reaches the torso, the person suffers gastrointestinal issues and, eventually, respiratory failure. An increased risk of this problem was detected during the flu season (August through December), but it was only two additional cases of GBS per one million vaccines. Vaccines for MMR, human papillomavirus (HPV), pneumococcal, varicella, and many other diseases do not have a statistical increase associated with GBS.

One fear associated with vaccine safety does have some merit, in that vaccines are thought to increase a variety of chronic autoimmune diseases. Some studies suggest a connection between self-antigens and overactive autoimmune responses when the vaccine enters a person's body and elicits an autobody response. This connection may predispose a child to type 1 diabetes and multiple sclerosis. Several epidemiologic studies have led researchers to conclude that there is no definitive link.

Scientists have seen an alarming increase in autoimmune diseases, primarily type 1 diabetes, since the vaccination schedule was updated in 2014, with approximately fifteen injections by age twelve years. Other autoimmune concerns are linked to the vaccine for human papillomavirus (HPV) infection, even though several significant European studies have not substantiated any adverse events. Researchers conducted a study in Denmark and Sweden to analyze over 690,000 participants who received the HPV vaccine. They concluded that there was no causal association with an autoimmune diagnosis.

Having too many vaccinations administered too soon is cited as the most significant barrier to vaccination compliance. This situation is perplexing because although the health-care community generally supports vaccinations, vaccinations may also increase autoimmune illnesses and nonspecific syndromes. A child in the United States can receive ten vaccines against fourteen diseases, all in the first few years of life. Many parents are concerned that so many vaccinations overwhelm the immature immune system. The vaccination schedule set by the CDC is said to have been developed to ensure that children get the best protection during the early stages of development

The debate on vaccine safety is ongoing and is often an emotional rather than rational consideration. Unsubstantiated media campaigns, celebrity endorsements, and biased research studies exacerbate the lack of faith in vaccinations. The anti-vaccination faction believes that greed on the part of pharmaceutical companies and corrupt government officials are using vaccination as a moneymaking scheme. There are studies that support both beliefs. Although there is statistical evidence that many diseases are reduced with vaccination, there remains a questionable concern about the impact vaccinations have on the long-term immunity responses of children. Mistrust and misinformation about the MMR vaccine's safety continue to overshadow the decisions of many parents to vaccinate their children. The security of the current vaccines in the United States supports the use of the MMR to reduce and potentially eliminate measles as a vaccine-preventable infection.

Vaccine Schedule

The future of vaccine safety is an app available through the CDC called the CDC Vaccine Schedules App for Health Care Providers. This app can be downloaded to a smartphone or tablet. It provides the current 2020 schedule and footnotes and looks similar to a printed schedule that is updated yearly. Providers can locate vaccines, dosages, and timing in a few clicks. The app can also develop a catch-up schedule, identify any contraindications, and highlight appropriate precautions. Future plans for the application include patient education flyers and hyperlinks for vaccine manufacturing tracking. The CDC is currently evaluating schedule changes to include the COVID-19 vaccines.

VACCINES AND AUTISM RESEARCH

The most current research trend is to examine the association between autism and the number of vaccinations children are scheduled to receive. According to the CDC, children received ten injections before being enrolled in a public school in the United States in 1983, at which time the rate of autism was 1 in 10,000. Today, children receive up to twenty-four vaccines before their first birthday, and by the time they enter public schools, they could have received as many as thirty-six. The rate of autistic children also has risen to 1 in 150 births. The medical community has not provided a conclusive reason for this alarming rise in autistic children. Some members of the medical community refer to genetics, but geneticists do not support this theory. Genetic disorders do not suddenly increase without some type of environmental trigger. Others point to better diagnostic testing; yet autism is based on a spectrum of symptoms, and the official criteria for determination have become more restrictive.

Many parents and pediatricians have voiced concerns over the increase in vaccinations. Dr. Russell Blaylock, a retired neurosurgeon, states that vaccinations elevate inflammatory cytokines, which are proteins secreted by the immune system that mediate the inflammatory cascade and regulate any response to disease or infection. The cytokine role is dichotomous; some cytokines perpetuate an appropriate immune response, while others cause autoimmune destruction. Studies have revealed elevated inflammatory cytokines present in autistic brain tissues, even up to forty-four years of age. Researchers subsequently suggest that the immune activation response to vaccination is extensive and can persist for decades. The discovery that those autistic children have elevated serum (blood) cytokine levels leads some people to conclude that vaccinations are the culprit in causing autism.

A preexisting dysfunction of the immune system has been found to engage the autism cascade with early and numerous vaccinations. Since the vaccine is different from a naturally acquired infection, the brain has a sustained immune response. Subsequent treatment elevates this response with each injection. The immune system is quickly activated and destroys the disease with naturally occurring conditions, as the immune system deactivates and recovers from the event after attacking and destroying the invader. However, vaccinations do not follow this natural pattern; vaccine-triggered immunity causes the immune system to stay at an elevated response for up to six months, causing global activation of the brain's inflammatory cells. This process could explain the extensive brain damage seen with autistic children.

The maturation of the developing child's brain is highly susceptible to the inflammatory response of vaccines. This response produces inflammation specific to the brain and targets cognitive and psychomotor skills. Excessive vaccination increases this risk and can be a factor leading to autism or other cognitive deficits. Research continues to address the possible (or probable) relationship between the MMR vaccine and the incidence of autism. Future research will need to follow stringent and ethical protocols to protect the most vulnerable members of our society—our children.

Drs. Frank DeStefano, Cristofer Price, and Eric S. Weintraub (2013) published a study in the *Journal of Pediatrics* that indicated no relationship between vaccines and children with autism spectrum disorder (ASD). The researchers used a case-control study conducted in a separately managed care organization that included 256 children with ASD and 752 children in the control group. The study concluded that children do not have an increased risk of developing ASD from the vaccines or components.

The link between autism and the mercury-based preservative thimerosal has been discredited. Nine CDC-funded or CDC-conducted studies found no connection between thimerosal-containing vaccines and ASD or the MMR vaccine. Thimerosal was removed from all childhood vaccines in the United States between the years 1999 and 2001. The only exception was some multidose influenza vaccines, but the amount has been substantially reduced; it is now listed as a trace amount.

Jain, Marshall, and Buikema (2015) published the most extensive study on vaccines and autism in the *Journal of American Medical Association*. The study included medical records of over 95,000 children who had an increased risk for autism or had an older sibling that had already been diagnosed with autism. The study concluded that receiving the MMR vaccine did not increase the risk of getting autism. Science continues to address this issue with the same results. The MMR vaccine protects children from contracting measles and is considered safe by multiple health-care organizations. Vaccine fears can only be addressed by providing education to parents and the general public that is transparent and evidence based.

BIOMEDICAL RESEARCH

Biomedical research encompasses a broad scope of medical science that seeks to prevent and treat diseases in animals and humans. This branch of science investigates the causes of conditions and the biological process that occurs from the disease. The purpose of this field of study is to develop effective treatments and, ultimately, cures. Animals are used in the research process to learn about the actual disease progression and ensure that new medical treatments are safe for humans. This specific research form is needed to identify how the body will react to novel diagnostic tools or therapeutic strategies.

Biomedical science and research have advanced an understanding of the intricate relationships between diseases and the immune system. The Institute of Biomedical Science was founded in the United Kingdom in the early 1900s. This prominent institute regularly supports research and publishes medical breakthroughs and diagnostic testing. Penicillin was a significant innovation discovered by the Scottish scientist Alexander Fleming in 1928. Additional antibiotics entered the health-care industry based on his work, which successfully decreased deaths worldwide. Animal research led to positive bone marrow transplants in mice after World War II. Subsequent human trials have established this treatment as safe, and it has been held responsible for saving hundreds of lives. Dr. Jonas Salk began innovations for a killed-virus polio vaccine. After testing the vaccine on over one million Canadian, American, and Finnish children in 1954, the vaccine was declared safe for the general public. The 1960s saw the MMR vaccine's invention by Dr. John Enders and his colleagues from the Edmonston B strain of measles.

Biomedical research has advanced understanding of the human genome over the past few decades. These scientific advancements are grounded in a randomized controlled study that manifests significant financial commitments and time. Today, many researchers devote their efforts to a faster and less expensive method of inquiry. This methodology uses the frameworks of meta-analyses and systematic reviews instead of clinical research. Over the past few years, the percentage of randomized controlled trials in these frameworks has been substantially less than synthetic studies using computer models. Synthetic studies are less time-consuming and are more cost-effective. As computer technology continues to expand and evolve artificial intelligence, this trend will become even more popular.

One exciting outcome of biomedical research is the development of an alternative to traditional vaccinations. One option of this type is a one-centimeter topical patch, called a *microarray patch*, that resembles a sticker. The patch has minute conical microneedles containing the vaccine in a polymer and sugar solution so that the vaccination is easily absorbed into the skin within minutes. There are many advantages to the patch vaccination method, especially in developing countries. The patches are easy to store and transport. They do not react to temperature shifts or require refrigeration like a traditional vaccine. Minimal training is necessary to administer the patch. The patches can be discarded in a regular waste receptacle after the person receives the vaccination. And the patches do not cause any pain or anxiety as opposed to receiving a shot. Dr. James Goodson, an epidemiologist with the Global Immunization Division of the CDC, expressed hope that this new tool could reach children in remote areas worldwide. Georgia Tech and the CDC collaborated on a study on microneedle patches and immune responses using rhesus macaques in 2012. The investigation led the scientist to conclude that the patches were beneficial and did not carry any side effects. Human clinical trials began in 2017 but failed to produce sufficient antibodies. However, the vaccination patch is still under scrutiny by the WHO and the CDC as a potential method of vaccination delivery.

The microarray patches are being examined for distribution in the African Region by government officials and the WHO. Many barriers would be overcome with the use of vaccination patches versus the traditional vaccination injection. The thermostability of the MMR patch allows transport to the dissolute areas of the country. The ease of application allows self-administration or use by a layperson. There is no need for medical supplies, syringes, needles, or a plan to dispose of the equipment. The used patch is considered nonmedical waste and will not harm the environment. A final advantage is a reduced need for supply chain requirements and cargo weight. It is predicted that once the patch has been implemented, the vaccine hesitancy in Africa will be reduced so that MMR vaccine compliance will improve.

Another futuristic vaccine delivery method is the dry powder measles vaccine (PMV), administered by an inhaler. The ClinicalTrials.gov website reported in 2018 that Phase I, an open-label randomized study for healthy adults, began in collaboration with the Serum Institute of India and the University of Colorado. The investigation is ongoing, but the researchers are optimistic about a favorable outcome. There are multiple measles inquires currently undergoing clinical trials. One study has led investigators to evaluate the administration of one dose of the MMR vaccine at four months of age instead of the traditional dose between nine months and one year. The goal is to enroll at least 3,750 children in the developing countries of Burkina Faso and Guinea-Bissau. Another study that began in 2017 in India compares two different measles vaccination schedules for infants. Infants receive protective antibodies from their mothers, and it is proposed the seroconversion with measles vaccination is ineffective for at least the first nine months of life. However, preliminary studies indicate that maternal antibodies are lost at six months. This study is a randomized controlled trial comparing the current schedule and a proposed schedule with earlier inoculation. A similar study was completed in 2008 with the data supporting the idea that the MMR vaccine not only prevents death in children under the age of five but reduces deaths from secondary infections. Multiple research studies on measles can be accessed through the Good Clinical Practice Network at ichgcp.net. This web page lists active, recruiting, ongoing, and completed research. Over 150 studies are listed that directly address the multifaceted need to continue the exploration of measles.

THE WORLD HEALTH ORGANIZATION'S
GLOBAL INITIATIVE

The goal of the *Global Measles and Rubella Strategic Plan, 2012–2020*, postulates that evidence supports a universal approach to protecting children and the general public from this highly contagious disease. Proponents of this strategic plan regard the MMR vaccine as the most cost-effective tool for public health to reduce the rate of measles cases. The executive summary builds on previous successes of measles control that reduced deaths by 74 percent globally from 2000 to 2010. The strategies address five core components: (1) high levels of vaccination compliance with the two-dose MMR vaccine, (2) effective surveillance programs, (3) preparedness for outbreaks, (4) communication with the general public to encourage participation with immunizations, and (5) continued research for improving vaccination and diagnostics.

The WHO partnered with the American Red Cross, the United Nations Foundation, the CDC, and United Nations Children's Fund (UNICEF) and launched a worldwide measles and rubella inoculation initiative in response to the global epidemic of measles. This initiative is in response to the three goals established toward eradicating measles in all nations. The first goal is that 90 percent of all children will receive their initial vaccination of MMR. The second goal is to reduce the annual incidence of measles to less than five cases per million. The third goal is to reduce measles-induced mortality by 95 percent by 2020. The organizations know that children must be vaccinated to achieve these lofty goals or outbreaks will occur, and measles will remain an endemic disease in many countries. Without inoculating most children, measles has the potential of a resurgence in countries where the disease was once eradicated, such as the United States.

Significant gains were achieved by the *Global Measles and Rubella Strategic Plan, 2012–2020*, and the necessary strategies were achievable: However, the plan did not have adequate support from many countries, and suboptimal funding further hampered the effort. It is suggested that those additional resources were needed to strengthen the immunization protocols leading to the achievement of the vaccination goals. Programs that supported mandated coverage for entry into schools and improved vaccination documentation were identified as achievable goals. The review of this strategic plan for 2020 goals is lofty and currently unmet, but redirecting the focus on improving existing immunization systems may increase vaccination rates and allow future success to build on current programs.

The WHO estimates that 5 percent of all deaths of children under the age of five in developing countries are from measles. This statistic relates directly to the United Nation's Millennium Development Goal 4 (MDG4): reducing childhood mortality by two-thirds. The United Nations uses the WHO's statistics of routine measles vaccination as an indicator of potential childhood mortality. Deaths caused by measles are preventable with inexpensive vaccines, and this fact makes it possible to reduce childhood mortality.

Worldwide, measles cases are climbing: In 2018, nearly 360,000 cases were recorded worldwide. The WHO reported 430,000 cases for 2019, with over 200,000 deaths recorded; most deaths were children under five years old. The WHO and UNICEF issued an emergency call to action for their global immunization partners on November 6, 2020. The partners include the American Red Cross, the United Nations Foundation, the CDC, the Bill and Melinda Gates Foundation, and others. The call to action is in response to the current coronavirus pandemic, which has shifted the world's attention and resulted in decreased efforts to maintain immunization campaigns. Strained health systems are overwhelmed and unprepared to fight the coronavirus and thus reduce the resources available to continue immunization campaigns for measles. At the emergency meeting, the *Measles & Rubella Strategic Framework 2021–2030* was developed to bolster the current delivery policies for all vaccines and reduce ineffective responses to outbreaks. However, this daunting task needs sustainable funding to be successful.

The Vaccine Alliance is the source of a large percentage of the funding for routine immunizations in developing countries. It also works independently to target children whose governments do not have an established vaccination program. The Vaccine Alliance has provided over 524 million children with immunizations from 2000 to 2018 through funded measles-rubella vaccination campaigns. The annual donor pledging conference for the Vaccine Alliance will be held virtually on April 8, 2022, from Germany. Supporters are hoping that the event will raise renewed interest in vaccination. The proposed goal for 2021 is $7 billion, earmarked to vaccinate 300 million children from 2021 to 2025. The United Kingdom International Development Secretary, Alok Sharma, is concerned that measles kills thousands of children from vaccine-preventable infections.

Inequalities of routine vaccination programs hinder the global initiative for measles vaccination. Despite global progress between 2000 and 2019, coverage for children living in certain countries is at a much lower ratio. Between 2010 and 2019, there was substantially slower progress in providing the MMR vaccine. The December 2020 issue of the *Nature Research Journal* included the report that as the Global Vaccine Action Plan (GVAP) compared the current first-dose MMR immunizations in low- to middle-income countries, the results were not favorable. Coverage in all countries within the study was stagnating or had declined since 2010. A noticeable slump was registered in 2020 as a result of the coronavirus pandemic. The

Equity Reference Group for Immunization echoes the need to continue vaccination efforts for those living in a rural environment and the urban poor. The group further advocates for health-care organizations to unite and develop sustainable goals. Today, many organizations have the same plan: to have every child receive the two-dose MMR vaccine. But all have different methods to pursue the dream.

MEASLES AND THE CORONAVIRUS PANDEMIC

Research predicts that the MMR vaccine will help protect some people from acquiring COVID-19 or reduce the symptoms of the virus. A study by Gold et al. published in the *American Society for Microbiology* (2020) analyzed MMR titers on fifty people who tested positive for COVID-19 and discovered that those with a higher level of measles antibodies (134 to 300 AU/ml) had less severe symptoms or no symptoms. Participants with moderate to severe symptoms had low measles antibody values (below 75 AU/ml). Scientists hypothesize that this results from the body's immune system recognizing the similarities in the two viruses.

A randomized, placebo-controlled two-phased research project began in August 2020 to assess the safety of the MMR vaccine and tolerance against the novel COVID-19. The Ain Shams University in Egypt started recruiting international participants in 2021 to explore the MMR vaccine's partial protection against COVID-19. The research hypothesis is that the measles vaccine may increase the immune system's response and improve its response to the coronavirus. Another hypothesis is that the coronavirus and measles have similar structural components, and cross-reactivity may exist. The reactivity may offer partial protection from COVID-19 and reduce the symptoms or shorten the length of time the person is infectious.

The CDC reports that as COVID-19 marches globally, over 117 million children may not receive their MMR vaccine. Too many countries have postponed vaccination campaigns to focus their human and financial resources on the COVID-19 pandemic. The pandemic requires the coordinated efforts of all to manufacture, supply, and vaccinate the world's population in response to the unprecedented event. At the same time, routine vaccinations must continue or a secondary pandemic may ensue.

After careful deliberation, the WHO has completed new guidelines to maintain immunization efforts. The guidelines allow countries that do not currently have active vaccine-preventable diseases, such as measles, to temporarily halt immunizations. This practice would enable areas where COVID-19 is an unacceptable high risk to funnel resources into vaccinating for this viral disease. The American Red Cross, the CDC, UNICEF, and the WHO all support this stance but recommend that all governments perform a risk-benefit analysis to determine the safest process for their populations.

There is much concern that the COVID-19 pandemic will result in a sharp rise in measles outbreaks. According to Gail McGovern, the president and chief executive officer of the American Red Cross, countries need to prioritize measles vaccination to mitigate the risk of outbreaks. More than 94 million people are currently at risk of missing their measles vaccines due to the ongoing COVID-19 pandemic. Measles is not constrained by borders or economics. Although the current pandemic requires a great deal of the existing health-care resources, the potential for another global disaster is possible if vaccinations are neglected. Measles is preventable; the MMR vaccine is a powerful, cost-effective, and safe vaccine. No one should be dying from this disease.

Case Studies

CASE 1: SABRINA HAS A BIRTHDAY

Sabrina was turning five years old. She and her mother celebrated by making chocolate and vanilla cupcakes with pink icing. Sabrina attended a private day care two days a week while her mother worked. She enjoyed her friends at day care and looked forward to having a birthday party with them, especially her best friend, Kailyn. Kailyn's favorite color was pink too. There would also be a pin the tail on the donkey game and treat bags.

Sabrina attended a private day care in an individual's home that was licensed by the state, and because it was a private business, it was not required to follow the current policies that mandated vaccinations for public schools. The day care administration provided weekly notifications to parents of any signs and symptoms of contagious illnesses. Kailyn's mother called the school early Monday and informed them that Kevin, Kailyn's two-year-old brother, had a high fever and a red rash, and Kailyn was not feeling well either. Kevin was taken to the pediatrician Monday morning and diagnosed with measles.

Sabrina and Kailyn attended the same church, and their families often got together for barbeques and pizza dinners. Kailyn and her family had met Sabrina's family at the local pizza restaurant for Sabrina's favorite food, pepperoni pizza, after church on the Sunday before her birthday. Everyone was laughing and having a great time, except for Kevin, who was a bit fussy during lunch. His cheeks seemed unusually pink, and he did not have his usual appetite. Since Kevin was not feeling well, the lunch was cut short. Kailyn hugged Sabrina goodbye and said, "See you tomorrow at school for your birthday party." Sabrina was so excited that she could hardly sleep Sunday night.

Sabrina arrived at the day care earlier than usual on Monday morning so that she and her mother could decorate the classroom. They tied balloons on the edge of a table at one corner of the room and arranged the cupcakes on a bright pink tablecloth. Sabrina and her mother placed the treat bags in the center of each child's desk. Sabrina's day care teacher had already planned to allow the pair to hang a pin the tail on the donkey game on the wall near the reading area. After decorating the classroom, they waited for the other children to arrive at the day care.

The children received birthday hats as they arrived at the day care and were excited to see the balloons and cupcakes! They were giddy with excitement and played together while they waited for everyone to arrive. Sabrina was sad to hear that Kailyn was ill and could not attend her party, but there was too much going on in the classroom to dampen the party atmosphere. The children exchanged party hats and began playing pin the tail on the donkey. Stephen won the game and received a unique treat bag for this accomplishment. After the game, the children ate their cupcakes and began their regular activities.

Monday afternoon, the day care notified the children's parents that a sibling of one of the students had measles. Sabrina's mother called Sabrina's pediatrician after being notified by the day care. Sabrina had not received the MMR vaccine as recommended by her pediatrician due to the family's religious beliefs. The triage nurse at the physician's office asked a few questions about Sabrina's current physical condition.

The nurse asked, "Does Sabrina have any cold symptoms?" The symptoms of measles often begin like a typical cold or the flu. As discussed in chapter 4, the symptoms include a cough, coryza (runny nose), and conjunctivitis (inflamed eyes). Even though Sabrina did not exhibit any symptoms, the nurse strongly encouraged Sabrina's mother to keep her away from other children for the next few days and to call back with any concerns.

Four days later, Sabrina had a dry hacking cough, runny nose, and reddened eyes. She also had flushed cheeks and a fever of 101 degrees. Her mother called the pediatrician again and was instructed to give Sabrina over-the-counter medication to reduce her fever and body aches. Two days later, Sabrina had a reddish-brown rash on her face. Calamine lotion helped relieve the intense itching sensation.

Sabrina had been exposed to measles from Kevin and Kailyn and now exhibited the classic symptoms of the virus. Sabrina's mother called the pediatrician once again for the advice. The physician used telemedicine to visualize Sabrina's rash and asked several questions, including, "What is her current temperature?" When Sabrina's mother responded with the details of her condition, the physician stated she had measles.

Analysis

Measles is a highly contagious virus found in the mucus membranes of the nose and throat. It is spread through the air when someone who has the virus coughs or sneezes. The aerosolized virus can travel up to two feet away and can also live on surfaces for approximately two hours. Sharing a drink or kissing a contagious person can also spread this disease. Ninety percent of unvaccinated peopled who come into contact with others suffering from measles (even before symptoms manifest) will contract the virus. An infected child attending a day care facility during the contagious period can infect all the children and staff who have not been vaccinated because they can be contagious for several days before the appearance of any symptoms.

Doctors recommend that a child diagnosed with measles get plenty of rest and fluids for the general flu-like symptoms. Frequent cool baths may help to control the discomfort of a fever, which often spikes in the afternoons. Over-the-counter nonaspirin antipyretics (fever reducers) help prevent the fever and reduce the risk of febrile seizures. Aspirin-containing medications are never recommended for viral illnesses because they have been linked to Reye's syndrome. Reye's syndrome is a rare but severe complication associated with taking aspirin. The syndrome causes swelling of the brain (encephalitis) and liver. Symptoms include gastrointestinal, respiratory, and neurological concerns that require emergency treatment, 40 percent of children with this disorder will die. Having a viral infection increases the risk for this disorder.

Most children with measles will be ill for approximately two weeks and experience general malaise, but they will recover without any permanent side effects and can be treated with over-the-counter medications. Children with measles should be isolated and have no minimal interaction with unvaccinated children and adults during the contagious period; this is especially true for those with weakened immune systems and pregnant women. The Centers for Disease Control and Prevention (CDC) recommends that parents seek medical treatment if any of the symptoms become severe, such as a fever (over 103 degree Fahrenheit) that does not respond to antipyretics, or if the child's overall condition worsens.

CASE 2: SARAH IS HAVING A BABY

Sarah and her husband, John, had been trying for the past year to get pregnant. They just received confirmation from Sarah's primary care doctor that she was six weeks pregnant! Sarah was prescribed prenatal vitamins and given a referral to see an obstetrician the next week. John was able to take a vacation day and attended the initial appointment with Sarah. Both wanted to keep their baby news a secret until they saw the obstetrician.

Their appointment was at nine o'clock on Tuesday morning. Sarah and John were both dressed and ready to go early and waited anxiously after having breakfast. The drive to the doctor's office was quiet and seemed to take a very long time. Finally, they arrived and started completing the new patient documentation; it was six detailed medical information pages. They only had to wait a few minutes after completing the paperwork to be escorted into an examination room. They were both excited to begin this new adventure and welcome their baby into the world. The examination room had a poster on the wall that described fetal growth over the next nine months, and John was reading some of the information to Sarah when the doctor came into the room.

Dr. Carolyn Farrell had been a pediatrician for twelve years and greeted the couple with a smile and handshake. The physician began to review Sarah's medical history and asked about her mother's hypertension (high blood pressure) and her father's diabetes. When she reached the page that addressed childhood illnesses, Dr. Farrell furrowed her brows and asked Sarah about the items marked as unknown. Sarah was unaware of her immunization status with measles because her mother had passed away several years ago and her father was not able to address these questions.

Sarah was a teacher at an elementary school, and her job increased her risk of exposure to childhood diseases, such as measles. The physician wanted to evaluate Sarah's immunity status with a blood test. She explained that this blood test was called a titer and that it checked for antibodies in the blood that determined whether the person was immune to a specific disease, including measles. After examining Sarah, the nurse drew blood for the titer test, and an appointment was made for the following week to review the results.

The next week, Sarah went to her obstetrician's office alone to get the results. The physician entered the examination room and informed Sarah that her titer was positive.

Sarah asked, "What does a positive titer test mean?"

The doctor explained that a positive test indicated that Sarah was considered immune to the disease either by vaccination or from having measles. She could safely continue teaching during her pregnancy without being at risk of contracting the disease. Sarah called John and informed him of the test results. John had a few additional questions for the doctor. Dr. Farrell was happy to address his questions.

John asked whether a booster shot for measles was a good idea for Sarah since she worked with children from an Orthodox Jewish community. Many children within the Orthodox Jewish community do not get vaccinated for religious reasons. The physician explained that a booster shot was not generally recommended when the titer had a positive result. The positive result meant that Sarah had developed an immunity to measles, and even with direct exposure to a contagious child, Sarah only had a 3 percent chance of contracting the infection.

That night, Sarah and John invited family and friends to a cookout at their home. John grilled steaks, and Sarah made her famous potato salad and chocolate cake. Everyone was having a great time! Before dessert, John stood behind Sarah's chair and said he had a big announcement: he and Sarah were having a baby. The entire group cheered and offered their congratulations.

Analysis

Women who live in the United States and plan to become pregnant should talk with their physicians about the risk of contracting measles, especially if they live in an area currently experiencing an outbreak. The physician can perform a blood test, known as a *titer*, to confirm immunity. If the test results are positive, the risk of contracting measles during pregnancy is less than 3 percent. If the test results are negative, the pregnant woman should not receive the MMR vaccine and not be exposed to anyone with a confirmed measles case.

Pregnancy reduces the immune system's efficiency, thereby increasing the potential for becoming infected with many illnesses, including measles. It is strongly encouraged for a woman to have a prepregnancy consultation with her obstetrician for a complete physical and health history. This consultation will include a review of all childhood illnesses and the woman's immune status. Vaccinations are lab tests that can be ordered by the physician. It is recommended that the woman obtain all vaccinations at least thirty days before trying to conceive. Chapter 9 explores the issues and controversies that are associated with measles and pregnancy.

If the woman is unvaccinated and contracts measles during pregnancy, the plan of care is the same as for other adults. Care includes supportive therapy based on her symptoms. Currently, there are no antiviral medications available that can be administered during pregnancy. Due to the potential complications, the pregnancy is considered high risk and requires diligent monitoring, especially for lung functionality.

CASE 3: JOHN IS A TRAVELING MAN

John was a regional sales manager for a retail clothing chain. He often traveled for his job all over the United States every week. Last year, he traveled 212 days to assess current merchandise and coordinate new purchases with the fifty stores that he oversees. After thirteen years, he still loved his job, but traveling so often and being away from his wife and daughter was stressful. He and his wife, Courtney, had been married for six years, and they had one daughter, Chelsea, who was five years old and his greatest joy.

For a conference, John's travel itinerary for the upcoming week had him traveling to San Diego, California. On Monday, before the trip, Chelsea had a playdate with a child in the neighborhood. The child's family also belonged to the same church as John and Courtney. The children played on the patio with Play-Doh and completed a puzzle. They had homemade cookies and juice just before the child went home with his mother. John enjoyed being home to see his daughter playing with a friend.

The following morning, John packed his suitcase and had breakfast with his family. The conversation bounced back and forth between Courtney and Chelsea as they discussed plans for a trip to the zoo with a group of friends later that week. John left for the airport shortly after breakfast and later called his wife after checking into his hotel room in California. Everything at home was good, but they missed him.

On Thursday, John was informed by his wife that the child who had played with Chelsea had been diagnosed with measles. The child had a red rash and fever. Her pediatrician had confirmed the diagnosis of measles. John had never had measles but was inoculated as a child with the MMR vaccine in 1964. The child had been contagious four days before the appearance of the rash and definitely exposed John to the virus. John had no symptoms and did not feel even the least bit ill. That evening, in the hotel room, he googled "exposure to measles." The internet offered a plethora of information on measles; some sites provided legitimate medical advice, and others were highly questionable. One site from a reputable medical organization emphasized the need for having the two-dose vaccination series. Only having one dose offered some protection, but with the second dose, a person achieves close to 100 percent protection.

John was concerned about the potential of contracting measles and spreading this virus to others. He contacted his primary care physician, Dr. Scott, and arranged for a phone conference.

"I have been exposed to a child that has a confirmed case of measles," John informed Dr. Scott. "Currently, I am traveling for my job and concerned with getting sick and exposing others to the illness." Then John asked, "What is the best course of action?"

Dr. Scott reviewed John's medical records, and it confirmed that John had received one of the two-dose MMR vaccinations; however, it was documented in the year 1964. During the years 1963–1967, there were some vaccines produced with a killed virus. This type of vaccination did not provide immunity for measles. Dr. Scott arranged for John to have a titer drawn (blood test) to assess his immunity status.

"I am recommending that you receive an additional MMR vaccine as soon as possible," Dr. Scott said. "I also want to draw blood to check your immunity status before you travel home."

"That sounds like a reasonable plan," John replied. "There is a laboratory near the convention center."

Dr. Scott advised John to remain isolated from others, as measles can be spread before symptoms appear. In fact, a contagious person can spread measles up to four days before they develop a rash. John had his blood work drawn that afternoon and received the results two days later. John's titer showed that he had immunity from measles. However, since he had only received one dose of the MMR vaccine, Dr. Scott recommended that John receive a booster vaccination. John traveled back home and made an appointment to receive his second MMR vaccine.

Analysis

John's risk for contracting measles with one vaccination is 95 percent, but with a second confirmed MMR injection, he has a 97 percent protection rate. What makes John susceptible to contracting measles is the year of vaccination. From 1963 to 1967, an ineffective version of the measles vaccine was manufactured and distributed throughout the United States. This version of the vaccine contained a "killed" virus, not the live-attenuated virus that has effectively protected against measles since 1963. John did not know which version he received in 1964, and it was better to be cautious and have a titer drawn and receive an additional MMR vaccine.

Measles is one of the most contagious viruses. The average person can expose twelve to eighteen people to the virus and has a 90 percent chance of infecting susceptible individuals. Susceptible individuals include unvaccinated children and adults, pregnant women, and anyone who is immunocompromised. The CDC recommends that people not board a plane with a fever, rash, or a confirmed measles diagnosis. Flying on a commercial flight increases the likelihood of being exposed to measles via aerosolized mucus droplets. The close proximity of individuals on the plane increases this exposure. The virus is found in the secretions of the mouth and throat and can be transmitted in the respiratory droplets of a cough or sneeze. The droplets can travel up to two feet and remain contagious on a surface for approximately two hours. No studies have linked the spread of measles through the airplane's air filtration system.

CASE 4: NICOLE AND CHRISTOPHER ARE HONEYMOONING ABROAD

Nicole and her fiancé, Christopher, were planning their dream wedding at an outdoor garden venue at a Southern plantation in Georgia. Their marriage was ten months away, and they had many details to consider.

Nicole had not even purchased the main component, her wedding dress. She had tried on a few at a local boutique, but nothing seemed to have the Southern charm she was searching to achieve.

Over the next few months, Nicole decided that the flowers would be magnolias and pink roses with natural foliage as an accent. The couple selected their favorite local restaurant to cater the wedding, and the menu was upscale barbeque. The venue had approved the usage of a large smoker on the premises. To continue the Southern wedding theme, lanterns would be hung from the large oak trees on the property, and hay bales covered in buffalo print blankets would provide extra seating. Everything seemed to be on track for the wedding, but the honeymoon proved to be a challenge.

Nicole and her fiancé were both avid photographers and dreamed of going on a photography safari in Kenya. The wedding was only a few months away, and they were unsure whether that was enough time to book the honeymoon. The Republic of Kenya—and many other regions in Africa—was currently experiencing a measles outbreak. The Ministry of Health attributed this to resistance to vaccination by religious groups and disruption in vaccination manufacturing. A traveler advisory had been issued for anyone traveling to the country. This advisory required people older than twelve years of age to provide evidence of immunity by providing proof that they had had the two-dose MMR vaccine or naturally acquired measles.

The couple made an appointment with a local travel agency. The agent assisted them with making the reservations, obtaining their passports, and completing the medical requirements for the international trip. One of the documents that the couple had to complete was about their immunity status for measles. The travel agent steered the couple to the CDC's travel vaccine assessment tool to assess their need for a measles vaccine. This tool asked a few simple questions and then provided a recommendation for the travelers.

Analysis

Nicole received two doses of the MMR vaccine during childhood and is considered to have 97 percent protection against measles. Christopher does not know whether he received the MMR vaccination during childhood or had measles, as both of his parents are deceased. For Nicole, the CDC considers her protected for life from measles. However, recent studies suggest that receiving an additional vaccination is prudent when traveling to areas, like Africa, with a current outbreak. Nicole contacted her physician to obtain the injection before her wedding.

Christopher was asked to complete additional questions because he was unable to provide evidence of immunity or documentation of having the MMR vaccine. The CDC recommended that he get two doses of the MMR vaccine with specific qualifiers. The two doses must be separated by 28 days and at least two weeks before departure. Christopher immediately contacted his physician, who suggested that a titer be drawn to assess his immunity status. The titer results were negative for measles immunity, and he received his first dose of the MMR vaccine. The second vaccination was scheduled a month before his wedding and within the CDC's guidelines. After receiving the second MMR injection, the CDC considers Christopher protected against measles for life.

Most measles cases in the United States are from international travelers entering the states or traveling to an area with a current outbreak or epidemic; this is the case for most of Africa. Africa is one of two continents that are currently experiencing a devastating measles outbreak. According to the World Health Organization (WHO), as of September 2019, over 44 percent of confirmed measles cases are in Africa. Measles is the leading cause of death among young children under the age of five in Africa. Reportedly, the current dynamics are a product of inadequate health-care infrastructure and the lack of government funding for vaccination.

CASE 5: A NURSE DOES NOT FOLLOW PROTOCOL

Roger was a twenty-six-year-old homosexual man who had been in a committed relationship for eight years with Timothy. Roger had been diagnosed with human immunodeficiency virus (HIV) for six of those years and was compliant with all his HIV medications. During the Christmas holidays, Roger and Timothy traveled to Key West for vacation. Upon returning, Roger complained of flu-like symptoms. Timothy encouraged Roger to see their physician, but he kept postponing making the call.

The symptoms continued for several days, and Roger became short of breath when walking to the bathroom. At this time, Timothy insisted that Roger see the doctor. Roger went to the doctor's office the next day and was short of breath and sweaty when he finally sat down in the waiting room. He was so pale that the receptionist immediately notified the triage nurse. The nurse came to the waiting room, helped Roger into a wheelchair, and took him to an examination room to see the doctor. Upon entering the examination room, the doctor saw Roger struggling to breathe and informed the nurse to call an ambulance right away.

Roger was admitted directly to a progressive care unit in respiratory distress. He was given oxygen to help him breathe and placed in a room with airborne precautions. Airborne precautions are infection prevention measures that prevent aerosolized mucus droplets from traveling through the air and being inhaled by another person. Three common illnesses require a facility to initiate airborne precautions: varicella virus (chickenpox), mycobacterium tuberculosis (TB), and measles.

The physician ordered a chest x-ray to visualize the health of Roger's lungs. When the radiologist reviewed the x-rays, it was evident that Roger had pneumonia. At first, the physician believed that the pneumonia was the result of his HIV status, and he discussed the diagnosis with Roger and Timothy. After a lengthy discussion with the couple, the physician considered their recent travel to the Florida Keys a risk factor for measles exposure. This location was currently experiencing an outbreak. The outbreak had been linked to the large population of the HIV-positive residents and visitors. HIV increases the risk of contracting measles, even with vaccination.

Evelyn was the nurse assigned to Roger in the hospital unit. She had been a nurse for ten years but was feeling overwhelmed with the long shifts. Roger's door had a notice that he was in airborne precautions, and there was a box attached to the door that held gloves, isolation gowns, and masks. When this is posted on a patient's door, everyone who enters the room must wear the personal protection equipment (PPE), per hospital protocol.

Evelyn was at the end of her shift and in a hurry. She did not put on the PPE when she entered the room to complete Roger's admission paperwork. The hospital notified Evelyn a few days later that Roger had measles. Measles is an acute respiratory illness that is spread by respiratory droplets. People with HIV are considered immunocompromised and may not develop the typical symptoms, like a rash.

Analysis

Health-care facilities have policies that address the safety of both the patient and the employees. These policies provide procedures that address strict precautions for isolating patients who present with potentially contagious symptoms. All HIV patients presenting with respiratory symptoms are included in this definition and are admitted with airborne precautions.

Airborne precautions require health-care personnel to wear gowns and gloves to protect their hands and clothing from being exposed to airborne droplets. Goggles and face shields protect the eyes and face from contamination. Health-care personnel must use unique masks, called respirators (N95 respirators), when they are within the room. The respiratory masks filter particles that are one micron in size and have a 95 percent filter efficiency with a proper facial seal.

The pathogenicity of measles is linked to the immune system of an infected individual. Most cases of measles are self-limiting, except for the immunocompromised. Individuals that are diagnosed with HIV and currently taking immunosuppressive drugs have increased risk of severe respiratory and neurological complications. Measles causes generalized immune dysfunction and life-threatening immunosuppression when combined with HIV medications.

Because measles is a virus that reproduces in the respiratory tract, health-care personnel must follow the guidelines to prevent exposure to the virus. A person with measles can spread the virus via a cough or sneeze up to two feet away. The aerosolized droplets can also live on surfaces for at least two hours. When a nurse does not follow the guidelines for airborne precautions, she puts her health and the health of those around her in jeopardy by not wearing a respiratory mask while in the patient's room. The nurse could also be at risk for disciplinary actions for not adhering to the facility's guidelines.

Glossary

Agglutination
Clumping of particles.

Alveoli
Tiny air sacs that allow for the exchange of oxygen and carbon dioxide.

Anthrax
An infection caused by the bacteria *Bacillus anthracis*.

Antihistamine
A drug that provides relief from sneezing, nasal congestion, and allergies.

Antipyretics
A medication that reduces fever.

Anti-vaxxers
People that do not believe in vaccinations.

Asterixis
Hand flapping.

Attenuated
Weakened viruses used in the MMR vaccine.

Autism
A disorder that is characterized with poor communication and social interaction.

Biopsy
Examining tissue that has been removed from a person to discover the presence of disease.

Bronchitis
Inflammation of the bronchial tubes.

Brucellosis
An infection caused by bacteria.

Capsaicin
The chemical found in chili peppers.

Chemotaxis
The movement of an organism responding to chemicals.

Chemotherapy
The use of drugs to kill cancerous cells.

Confabulation
A memory disorder when a person gives false answers to fill in memory gaps.

Conjunctiva
The membrane that covers the inside of the eyelid and the front of the eye.

Conjunctivitis
Inflammation of the eye, commonly known as pink eye.

Contagious
Disease or infection that can spread from one person to another.

Corneal ulceration
An open sore on the cornea.

Coryza
Runny nose.

Croup
An infection in the upper airways that obstructs breathing. Croup has a distinctive bark-like cough.

Cytokines
Substances secreted by cells in the immune system that affect other cells.

Dengue fever
A mosquito-borne viral disease in tropical areas.

Divergence
The process of two species becoming a new organism.

Dysthymias
Irregular beating of the heart.

Edema
Swelling.

Encephalitis
Inflammation and swelling of the brain.

Endemic
A disease found among a geographical location.

Epidemic
The rapid spread of disease to people within a specific time period.

Epidemiologist
A scientist who studies diseases.

Excipients
An inactive substance that is a medium for other active ingredients.

Expressive aphasia
The inability to produce speech, verbal or written.

Febrile
Fever.

Gastrointestinal
The hollow tubule organs from the mouth to the anus.

Guillain-Barré syndrome (GBS)
Rare autoimmune disorder that damages the nerve cells.

Herd Immunity
When a large portion of the population is immune to a specific disease.

Holoendemic
When every person in a population is infected with a disease or illness.

Homeostasis
A relatively stable environment within the body.

Hyperendemic ocular trachoma
An ocular infection that causes visual impairment or blindness.

Hypertension
High blood pressure.

Hypothalamus
A small organ at the base of the brain that releases hormones and regulates the body temperature.

Idiopathic (or immune) thrombocytopenic purpura (ITP)
An immune disorder that results in the blood not clotting properly.

Immune amnesia
Severe suppression of the body's immune memory.

Immunity
The ability of a person to resist an infection or toxin with antibodies.

Immunosuppression
Suppression of the immune response to foreign particles or infections.

Isolation
The process of being set apart from others; being isolated.

Keratitis
Inflammation of the cornea. The cornea is a transparent membrane that covers the pupil and iris.

Keratomalacia
An eye disorder when the cornea gets cloudy and impairs vision.

Koplik's Spots
Spots inside the mouth in the buccal region that indicate the early phase of measles. The spots are bluish-white with red rings.

Laryngitis
Inflammation of the larynx (voice box). Symptoms include hoarseness or loss of voice.

Laryngotracheobronchitis
A respiratory infection caused by a virus; also known as croup.

Leukocytes
Cells that assist in identifying foreign particles and diseases.

Lingual
Related to speech or language.

Lymphadenopathy
Enlargement of the lymph glands.

Lysis
The breakdown of cells by rupturing the cell walls.

Maculopapular rash
A rash with raised and flat lesions that are usually red.

Malaise
General discomfort that is difficult to identify.

Morbillivirus
Virus that needs a host from the *Paramyxoviridae* family.

Myelin
The white insolating sheath that surrounds some nerve fibers.

Myocardial infarction
Damage to the cardiac muscle.

Neutrophil
A white blood cell.

Nonpharmaceutical
Interventions that a person can use to prevent or control an illness, such as isolation.

Opsonization
The mechanism when a pathogen is connected to an antibody at the cell's receptor sites.

Optic neuritis
Inflammation that damages the optic nerve.

Otitis media
Middle-ear infection.

Paramyxoviridae
A negative strand RNA virus that causes measles and respiratory tract infections.

Paraparesis
Partial paralysis of the legs.

Paraplegia
Paralysis of the lower body and legs.

Paresthesia
An abnormal sensation of the skin, such as tingling or numbness.

Pathogen
A virus, bacteria, or microorganism that can cause disease.

Pertussis
An extremely contagious respiratory infection; also known as whooping cough.

Petechiae
Small round spots on the skin from bleeding.

Phagocyte
A cell that destroys other cells or particles.

Photophobia
Extreme sensitivity to light.

Pneumonia
Inflammation of the lungs that may fill the air sacs with fluid.

Prophylaxis
Preventive health care.

Prosopagnosia
A neurological disorder that prevents a person from recognizing the faces of familiar people.

Pyrexia
Fever.

Quarantine
The period of time that people must isolate to prevent the spread of disease.

Receptive Aphasia
Difficulty understanding written or spoken language.

Retinopathy
A disease of the retina that may impair vision or cause blindness.

Rinderpest
Cattle plague or measles of cattle or buffalo.

Sclera
White outermost part of the eyeball.

Seizures
Uncontrolled electrical activity in the brain that causes abnormal thoughts and movements of the body.

Stimming
Abnormal body movements associated with autism.

Surveillance
A reporting system for suspected cases of a disease, such as measles.

Thrombocytopenia
A blood disorder where the platelet count is low, reducing the blood's ability to form a clot.

Titer
Blood test to discover antibody concentration.

Trypsin
Enzyme that helps digest protein.

Trypsinogen
Substance secreted by the pancreas that forms trypsin in the digestive tract.

Tussis
The act of coughing.

Urticaria
Swollen, pale red bumps on the skin that appear as a result of an allergen; also known as hiver.

Urticaria rash
A skin rash with pale red swollen areas.

Vesicular rash
A tapioca-like rash with blisters.

Xerophthalmia
Extreme dryness of the eyes.

Directory of Resources

BOOKS

Byrne, J., and J. Hays. (2021). *Epidemics and pandemics: From ancient plagues to modern-day threats.* Greenwood.

Colligan, L. (2011). *Measles and mumps.* Marshall Cavendish Benchmark.

Deer, B. (2020). *The doctor who fooled the world: Science, deception, and the war on vaccines.* Scribes Publications.

Rosaler, M. (2004). *Measles.* Rosen Publishing Group.

Wilfred, A. (2019). *Measles: Guide to symptoms, causes, diagnosis & treatment.* Independently published.

ORGANIZATIONS

Centers for Disease Control and Prevention (CDC)

1600 Clifton Rd

Atlanta, GA 30329

Cdc.gov

800-232-4636

National public health agency for the United States.

Measles & Rubella Initiative

Managed by the American Red Cross

2700 Southwest Fwy

Houston, TX 77098

800-733-2767

https://measlesrubellainitiative.org/

Global partnership for measles and rubella vaccination.

National Library of Medicine

8600 Rockville Pike

Bethesda, MD 20894

301-594-5983

888-346-3656

https://www.nlm.nih.gov/

The most extensive medical library in the United States with a vast collection of health-care-related topics.

Pan American Health Organization (PAHO)

525 23rd St NW

Washington, DC 20037

https://www.paho.org/en/topics/measles

International health-care organization for the Inter-American System that supports the health-care infrastructure and responds to emergencies.

World Health Organization (WHO)

20 Avenue Appia

1211 Geneva 27

Switzerland

Fax: 41 22 791 4894

International public health organization under the guidance of the United Nations.

WEBSITES

"Eliminating Measles and Rubella"—World Health Organization

https://www.who.int/westernpacific/activities/eliminating-measles-and
-rubella

Information about the WHO's efforts to eradicate measles globally.

"Measles"—Mayo Clinic

https://www.mayoclinic.org/diseases-conditions/measles/symptoms
-causes/syc-20374857

Information about the causes, symptoms, diagnosis, and treatment of measles from one of the United States' premier medical institutions.

"Measles"—MedlinePlus

https://medlineplus.gov/measles.html

Information on measles from a large web-based library of health information.

"Measles Elimination"—Centers for Disease Control and Prevention

https://www.cdc.gov/measles/elimination.html

Information on efforts to eradicate measles in the United States.

"Measles (Rubeola)"—Centers for Disease Control and Prevention

https://www.cdc.gov/measles/index.html

The CDC's homepage for measles information and resources.

"This Is How Easy It Is to Spread Measles"—National Foundation for Infectious Diseases

https://www.nfid.org/infectious-diseases/this-is-how-easy-it-is-to-spread
-measles/

A short animated video exploring the extreme transmissibility of measles.

Bibliography

American Cancer Society. (2019). Key statistics for childhood leukemia. https://www.cancer.org/cancer/leukemia-in-children/about/key-statistics.html

American Red Cross. (2020, November 12). Coronavirus slows measles prevention work around the globe. https://www.redcross.org/about-us/news-and-events/news/2020/coronavirus-slows-measles-prevention-work-around-the-globe.html

Bell, S., Clarke, R., Paterson, P., & Mounier-Jack, S. (2020, December 28). Parents' and guardians' views and experiences of accessing routine childhood vaccination during the coronavirus (COVID-19) pandemic: A mixed methods study in England. *PLoS ONE, 15*(12), e0244049. https://doi.org/10.1371/journal.pone.0244049

Bhaskaram, P. (1995). Measles & malnutrition. *Indian Journal of Medical Research, 102*, 195–199. https://pubmed.ncbi.nlm.nih.gov/8675238/

Biddlecombe, S. (2018, August 20). Feel lonely? There are 4 types of loneliness. Here's how to beat them. *Stylist*. https://www.stylist.co.uk/long-reads/how-to-deal-with-loneliness-types-emotional-situational-social-chronic/222923

Blach, C., Kaye, J., & Jick, H. (2003). MMR vaccine and idiopathic thrombocytopenic purpura. *British Journal of Clinical Pharmacology, 55*(1), 107–111. https://doi.org/10.1046/j.1365-2125.2003.01790.x

Capatides, C. (2016, March 18). 30 of Donald Trump's wildest quotes: On vaccinations. CBS Newshttps://www.cbsnews.com/pictures/wild-donald-trump-quotes/21/

Caspi, A., Harrington, H., Moffitt, T., Milne, B. J., & Poulton, R. (2006). Socially isolated children 20 years later: Risk of cardiovascular disease. *Archives of Pediatric Adolescent Medicine, 160*(8), 805–811. https://doi.org/10.1001/archpedi.160.8.805

Centers for Disease Control and Prevention. (2021a, August 10). Hand-washing: Clean hands save lives: When and how to wash your hands. https://www.cdc.gov/handwashing/when-how-handwashing.html

Centers for Disease Control and Prevention. (2021b, February 23). Immunization schedules: CDC Vaccine Schedules app for health care providers. https://www.cdc.gov/vaccines/schedules/hcp/schedule-app.html

Centers for Disease Control and Prevention. (2020a, November 5). Measles (rubeola): Complications of measles. https://www.cdc.gov/measles/symptoms/complications.html

Centers for Disease Control and Prevention. (2020b, November 5). Measles (rubeola): For public health professionals. https://www.cdc.gov/measles/stats-surv.html

Centers for Disease Control and Prevention. (2020c, November 5). Measles (rubeola): Genetic analysis of measles viruses. https://www.cdc.gov/measles/lab-tools/genetic-analysis.html

Centers for Disease Control, and Prevention. (2020d, November 5). Measles (rubeola): Signs and symptoms. https://www.cdc.gov/measles/symptoms/signs-symptoms.html

Centers for Disease Control and Prevention. (2014). *Manual for the surveillance of vaccine-preventable disease.* Centers for Disease Control and Prevention. https://www.cdc.gov/vaccines/pubs/surv-manual/index.html

Children's Hospital of Philadelphia. (n.d.). Idiopathic thrombocytopenic purpura (ITP) causes, symptoms, and treatment. https://www.chop.edu/conditions-diseases/idiopathic-thrombocytopenic-purpura-itp

Cleveland Clinic. (2017, March 1). What happens when your immune system gets stressed out? https://health.clevelandclinic.org/what-happens-when-your-immune-system-gets-stressed-out/

Coghlan, A. (2010, May 24). Banned: Doctor who linked vaccine with autism. https://www.newscientist.com/article/dn18954-banned-doctor-who-linked-mmr-vaccine- with-autism/

Curley, C. (2020, November 23). How the measles vaccine may help protect against COVID-19. Healthline. https://www.healthline.com/health-news/how-the-measles-vaccine-may-help-protect-against-covid-19

Dang, S. (2015, March 5). Six ways measles can affect the eyes. https://www.aao.org/eye-health/tips-prevention/six-ways-measles-can-affect-eyes-2

De Figueiredo, A., Simas, C., Karafilakis, E., Paterson, P., & Larson, H. (2020). Mapping global trends in vaccine confidence and investigation barriers to vaccine uptake: A large-scale retrospective temporal modelling study. *The Lancet.* https://doi.org/10.1016/S0140-6736(20)31558-0

Deer, B. (2020). *The doctor who fooled the world: Science, deception, and the war on vaccines.* Scribes Publications.

DeStefano, F., Bodenstab, H., & Offit, P. (2019). Principal controversies in vaccine safety in the United States. *Journal of Clinical Infectious Diseases, 69*(4), 726–731. https://doi.org/http://dx.doi.org/10.1093/cid/ciz135

DeStefano, F., Price, C., & Weintraub, E. (2013). Increasing exposure to antibody-stimulation proteins and polysaccharides in vaccines is not associated with risk of autism. *Journal of Pediatrics, 163*(2), 561–567. https://www.jpeds.com/article/S0022-3476(13)00144-3/pdf

Doane, L. D., & Adam, E. K. (2010). Loneliness and cortisol: Momentary, day-to-day, and trait association. *Psychoneuroendocrinology, 35*(3), 430–431. https://doi.org/10.1016/j.psyneuen.2009.08.005

Duflos, C., Troude, P., Strainchamps, D., Segouin, C., Loeart, D., & Mercier, G. (2020). Hospitalization for acute heart failure: The in-hospital care pathway predicts one-year readmission. *Scientific Reports, 10*, 10644. https://doi.org/10.1038/s41598-020-66788-y

Encephalitis Society. (2019). *After-effects of encephalitis.* https://www.encephalitis.info/pages/category/after-effects-of-encephalitis

Farber, M. (2020, November 12). *Measles case confirmed in child who may have exposed others at Washington State airport.* Fox News. https://www.foxnews.com/health/measles-case-child-washington-state-airport

Finnegan, G. (2019, November 4). EU commissioner: "I will always be a vaccine advocate." *Vaccines Today.* https://www.vaccinestoday.eu/stories/eu-commissioner-i-will-always-be-a-vaccine-advocate/

Frankel, G. (2004). Charismatic doctor at vortex of vaccine dispute. *The Washington Post.* https://www.washingtonpost.com/archive/politics/2004/07/11/charismatic-doctor-at-vortex-of-vaccine-dispute/09772e4c-c904-474c-92a1-9740e12dacb7/

Gallagher, G. (2020, November 12). *Measles killed 207K people in 2019 as cases hit 23-year high.* Healio. https://www.healio.com/news/infectious-disease/20201112/measles-killed-207k-people-in-2019-as-cases-hit-23year-high

Gastanaduy, P., Budd, J., Fisher, N., Redd, S., Fletcher, J., Miller, J., McFadden, D., Rota, J., Rota, P., Hickman, C., Fowler, B., & Tatham, L. (2016, October 6). A measles outbreak in an underimmunized Amish community in Ohio. *New England Journal of Medicine, 375*, 1343–1354. https://doi.org/10.1056/NEJMoa1602295

Gavi. The Vaccine Alliance (2022). Germany to co-host 2022 Gavi COVAX AMC Summit, pledges additional funding for COVID-10 vaccination in lower-income countries. https://www.gavi.org/news/media

-room/germany-co-host-2022-gavi-covax-amc-summit-pledges
-additional-funding-covid-19

Gessen, M. (2019, March 2). Why measles is a quintessential political issue of our time. *The New Yorker* https://www.newyorker.com/news /our-columnists/why-measles-is-a-quintessential-political-issue -of-our-time

Gilmour, J. (2019). Airline passenger spread measles to travelers on flight to San Francisco. *Sacramento Bee.* https://www.sacbee.com/news /california/article227261869.html

Gold, J., Baumgart, W., Okyay, R., Licht, W., Fidel, P., Novert, M., Tilley, L., Hurley, D., Rada., B., & Ashford, J. (2020, November/December). Analysis of measles-mumps-rubella (MMR) titers of recovered COVID-19 patients. *American Society for Microbiology, 11*(6), 1–10. https://doi.org/10.1128/mBio.02628-20

Good Clinical Practice Network. (2020, July 1). *Measles vaccine: Is there a protective role in COVID 19 pandemic?* https://ichgcp.net/clinical -trials-registry/NCT04445610

Gurhan, N., Beser, N., Polat, U., & Koc, M. (2019). Suicide risk and depression in individuals with chronic illness. *Community Mental Health Journal, 55,* 840–848. https://doi.org/10.1007/ s10597-019-00388-7

Hall, J., Lozano, M., Estrada-Petrocelli, L., Birring, S., & Turner, R. (2020, September). The present and future of cough counting tools. *Journal of Thoracic Disease, 12*(9), 5207–5223. https://doi.org/10.21037 /jtd-2020-icc-003

Handley, J. B. (2005). Autism: First person perspective: Rescuing a generation. Autism Advocate. https://www.autism-society.org/wp-content /uploads/2014/04/Rescuing-a-Generation.pdf

Hyman, M., (2018). *Food: What the heck should I eat?* Little, Brown, and Company.

I Vaccinate. (2019, May 8). A 5-month-old baby got the measles—Now her mom has a message for parents. https://ivaccinate.org/a-5-month -old-baby-got-the-measles-now-her-mom-has-a-message-for -parents/

Infectious Diseases Society of America. (2015, October 8). One in eight children at risk for measles. ScienceDaily. https://www.sciencedaily .com/releases/2015/10/151008142235.htm

Jain, A., Marshall, J., Buikema, A. (2015). Autism occurrence by MMR vaccine status among US children with older siblings with and without autism. *Journal of the American Medical Association.* 391(15). 1534-1540. doi:10.1001/jama.2015.3077

Khodabaklsh, M., Mehri, M., Ghorbani, F., & Feyzabadi, Z. (2016). Measles from the perspective of Rhazes and traditional Iranian medicine: A

narrative review. *International Journal of Pediatrics, 4*(10), 361–
3668. https://doi.org/10.22038/ijp.2016.7628

Kim, E. K. (2019, April 29). The classic "Brady Bunch" episode is suddenly
at the center of the measles vaccine debate. Today. https://www
.today.com/health/brady-bunch-episode-fueling-efforts-against
-measles-vaccine-t153029

Koh, H. K., & Gekkub, B. G. (2020). Measles as metaphor—What resurgence means for the future of immunization. *Jama, 323*(10), 914–
915. https://doi.org/10.1001/jama.2020.1372

Lacey, R., Kumari, M., & Bartley, M. (2014). Social isolation in childhood
and adult inflammation: Evidence from the National Child Development Study. *Science Direct, 50,* 85–94. https://doi.org/10.1016/j
.psyneuen.2014.08.007

Lane, L. (2019, June 2). Latest news about the measles outbreak, international travel, and preventative measures. Forbes. https://www.forbe
s.com/sites/lealane/2019/06/02/latest-news-about-the-measles
-outbreak-international-travel-and-preventative-measures/

Langgut, D., Cheddadi, R., & Sharon, G. (2021). Climate and environmental reconstruction of the Epipaleolithic Mediterranean Levant. *Science Direct, 270,* 107–170. https://www.sciencedirect.com/science
/article/abs/pii/S0277379121003772?dgcid=rss_sd_all

LaVito, A. (2019). Federal health officials urge some adults to get revaccinated against measles amid worst outbreak in 25 years. *CNBC
Health and Science.* https://www.cnbc.com/2019/04/30/us-health
-officials-urge-some-adults-to-get-vaccinated-against-measles
.html

Leppart, E. (2020, April 7). How sugar damages your immune system +
how to cut it out. Nutritional Weight & Wellness. https://www
.weightandwellness.com/resources/articles-and-videos/how-sugar
-damages-your-immune-system-how-cut-it-out/

Majumder, M. S., Cohn, E. L., Mekaru, S. R., Huston, J. E., & Brownstein,
J. S. (2015, May 15). Substandard vaccination compliance and the
2015 measles outbreak. *JAMA Pediatrics, 169*(5), 494–495. https://
doi.org/10.1001/jamapediatrics.2015.0384

Manhire, T. (2019). Oh great, New Zealand might have just given Disneyland
measles. *The Spinoff.* https://thespinoff.co.nz/science/25-08-2019/oh
-great-new-zealand-might-have-just-given-disneyland-measles

Manhire, T. (2019). Oh great, New Zealand might have just given Disneyland
measles. *The Spinoff.* https://thespinoff.co.nz/science/25-08-2019/oh
-great-new-zealand-might-have-just-given-disneyland-measles

Mayo Clinic. (2020, February). Optic neuritis. https://www.mayoclinic
.org/diseases-conditions/optic-neuritis/diagnosis-treatment/drc
-20354958

Mayo Clinic (2020). The not-so-sweet truth of added sugars. https://www
    .mayoclinichealthsystem.org/hometown-health/speaking-of
    -health/the-not-so-sweet-truth-of-added-sugars

Measles & Rubella Initiative. (2021). The anti-vaccination movement.
    https://measlesrubellainitiative.org/anti-vaccination-movement/

Measles & Rubella Initiative. (2020, November 11). COVID-19's impact
    on measles vaccination coverage. Centers for Disease Control and
    Prevention. https://www.cdc.gov/globalhealth/measles/news/covid
    -impact-on-measles-vaccination.html

Measles & Rubella Initiative. (2020). The measles & rubella initiative sup-
    ports the implementation of the Measles & Rubella Strategic
    Framework 2021–2030. https://measlesrubellainitiative.org/learn
    /the-solution/the-strategy/

Meira, I., Romano, T., Pires do Prado, H., Kruger, L., Pires, M., & da Con-
    ceiclio, P. (2019). Ketogenic diet and epilepsy: What we know so far.
    Frontiers in Neuroscience, 13. https://www.frontiersin.org/articles
    /10.3389/fnins.2019.00005/full

Michael, B., & Solomon, T. (2012). Seizures and encephalitis: Clinical fea-
    tures, management, and potential pathophysiologic mechanism.
    Epilepsia, 53(4), 63–71. https://doi.org/10.1111/j.1528-1167.2012
    .03615.x

Miller, E., Weight, P., Farrington, C., Andrews, N., Stowe, H., & Taylor, B.
    (2001). Idiopathic thrombocytopenic purpura and MMR vaccine.
    Archives of Disease in Childhood, 83(3), 227–229. http://dx.doi
    .org/10.1136/adc.84.3.227

Mina, M., Kula, T., Leng, Y., Li, M., de Vries, R., & Knip, M. (2019). Measles
    virus infection diminishes preexisting antibodies that offer protec-
    tion for other pathogens. *Science, 366*(6465), 599–606. https://doi
    .org/10.1126/science.aay6485

Ministry of Health. (2012). *Protecting children with cancer from measles.*
    Wellington: Ministry of Health. https://www.health.govt.nz/system
    /files/documents/publications/protecting-children-with-cancer
    -from-measles.pdf

Misra, U., Tan, C., & Kalita, J. (2008). Viral encephalitis and epilepsy. *Epilep-
    sia, 49*(6), 13–18. https://doi.org/10.1111/j.1528-1167.2008.01751.x

Mooney, Graham. (2011). Historical demography and epidemiology: The
    meta-narrative challenge. Oxford University Press.

Mor, G. (2020). Infection and pregnancy. https://mott.med.wayne.edu
    /infectionandpregnancy

Munoz-Alia, M., Muller, C., & Russell, S. (2017). Antigenic drift defines a
    new D4 subgenotype of measles virus. *Journal of Virology, 91*(11), 1.
    https://doi.org/10.1128/JVI.00209-17

Najera, R. F. (2019, March 12). Vitamin A and measles. College of Physicians of Philadelphia. https://www.historyofvaccines.org/content/blog/vitamin-a-measles

National Measles and Rubella Laboratory. (n.d.). WHO-accredited Canterbury Health Laboratories. Measles.co.nz/home

Nichols, E. M. (1979). Atypical measles syndrome: A continuing problem. *American Journal of Public Health, 69*(2), 160–162. https://doi.org/10.2105/AJPH.69.2.160

Njau, J., Janta, D., Stanescu, A. et al. (2019). *Assessment of economic burden of concurrent measles and rubella outbreaks, Romania, 2011–2012. Emerging Infectious Diseases, 25*(6), 1101–1109. https://doi.org/10.3201/eid2506.180339

No Isolation. (2019, April 29). Consequences of social isolation for children and adolescents. https://www.noisolation.com/global/research/consequences-of-social-isolation-for-children-and-adolescents/

Otterman, S. (2019, January 17). New York confronts its worst measles outbreak in decades. *The New York Times.* https://www.nytimes.com/2019/01/17/nyregion/measles-outbreak-jews-nyc.html

Palmer, A. (2019). Truth will prevail—1200 studies that refute vaccine claims [e-book]. Dukumen.Pub. https://dokumen.pub/truth-will-prevail-1200-studies-that-refute-vaccine-claims-26nbsped.html

Paul, I., Beiler, J., McMonagle, A., Shaffer, M., Duda, L., & Berlin, C. J. (2007). Effect of honey, dextromethorphan, and no treatment on nocturnal cough and sleep quality for coughing children and their parents. *Pediatric Adolescent Medicine, 161*(12), 1140–1146. http://dx.doi.org/10.1001/archpedi.161.12.1140

Paun, C. (2017, February 9). Trump offers vindication to vaccine skeptic doctor. Politico. https://www.politico.eu/article/disgraced-doctor-who-questioned-vaccine-safety-looks-to-trump-with-hope/

Perry, R., & Halsey, N. (2004). The clinical significance of measles: A review. *Journal of Infectious Diseases, 189*(1), S4–S16. https://doi.org/10.1086/377712

Petrova, V., Sawatsky, B., Han, A., Laksono, B., Walz, L., Parker, E. Pieper, K., Anderson, C., De Vries, R., Kellam, P., Messling, V., DeSwart, R., & Russell, C. (2019, November 1). Incomplete genetic reconstitution of B cell pools contributed to prolonged immunosuppression after measles. *Science Immunology, 4.* https://www.science.org/doi/10.1126/sciimmunol.aay6125

Pike, J., Leidner, A., & Gastanaduy, P. (2020). A review of measles outbreak cost estimated from the United States in the postelimination era (2004–2017): Estimates by perspective and cost type. *Clinical Infectious Diseases, 71,* 1568–1576. https://doi.org/10.1093/cid/ciaa070

Plaugic, L. (2015, April 27). Researchers are working on a patch that can vaccinate wearers against measles. The Verge. theverge.com/2015 /4/27/8504671/measles-vaccine-microneedle-patch-cdc

Rana, M. S., Alam, M. M., Ikram, A. et al. (2021). Emergence of measles during the COVID-19 pandemic threatens Pakistan's children and the wider region. *Natural Medicine, 27*, 1127–1128. https://doi.org /10.1038/s41591-021-01430-6

Rao, T. S. Sathyanarayana, & Andrade, C. (2011). The MMR vaccine and autism: Sensation, refutation, retraction, and fraud. *Indian Journal of Psychiatry, 53*(2), 95–96. https://doi.org/10.4103 /0019-5545.82529

Reliefweb. (2022). Germany to co-host 2022 Gavi COVAX AMC Summit, pledges additional funding for COVID-19 vaccination in lower-income countries. Press Release. https://reliefweb.int/report/world /germany-co-host-2022-gavi-covax-amc-summit-pledges -additional-funding-covid-19

Richardson, L., & Moss, W. (2020). Measles and rubella microarray array patches to increase vaccination coverage and achieve measles and rubella elimination in Africa. *Pan African Medical Journal, 35*(3). https://jhu.pure.elsevier.com/en/publications/measles-and -rubella-microarray-array-patches-to-increase-vaccinat

Ries, J. (2019, April 23). Vaccinated people can get measles, but this is why you need the shot. Healthline. https://www.healthline.com/health -news/yes-even-vaccinated-people-can-get-measles-heres-why -you-should-still-get-the-shot

Roberts, M. (2019, June 19). Vaccines: Low trust in vaccination "a global crisis." BBC News. https://www.bbc.com/news/health-48512923

Roser, M., Ritchie, H., & Dadonaite, B. (2019). Childhood and infant mortality. Our World in Data. https://ourworldindata.org/child -mortality

Rota, P., Brown, K., Mankertz, A., Santibanez, S., Shulga, S., Muller, C., Hubschen, J., Siqueira, M., Beirnes, J., & Ahmed, H. (2011). Global distribution of measles genotypes and measles molecular epidemiology. *Journal of Infectious Diseases, 204*(1), 514–523. https://doi .org/10.1093/infdis/jir118

Sbarra, A. et al. (2020). Mapping routine measles vaccination in low- and middle-income countries. *Nature, 589*, 415–419. https://doi.org /10.1038/s41586-020-03043-4

Schwartz, K. (2019, March 14). What you need to know about measles and airplanes. *New York Times.* https://www.nytimes.com/2019/03/14 /travel/measles-outbreak-airplanes-vaccines.html

Science Media Centre. (2019). Expert reaction to stud looking at vaccination policies and measles resurgence. https://www.sciencemediacentre

.org/expert-reaction-to-study-looking-at-vaccination-policies
-and-measles-resurgence/

Shanks, D. (2016). Pacific Island societies destabilised by infectious disease. *Journal of Military and Veterans' Health, 24*(4), 71–74. https://jmvh.org/article/pacific-island-societies-destabilised-by-infectious-diseases/

Shulman, S. T., Shulman, D. L., & Sims, R. H. (2009). The tragic 1824 journey of the Hawaiian king and queen to London: History of measles in Hawaii. *Pediatric Infectious Disease Journal, 28*(8), 728–733. https://doi.org/10.1097/INF.0b013e31819c9720

Sidhu, S. (2020, February 5). Global measles vaccination drive to protect up to 45 million children. UNICEF. https://www.unicef.org/press-releases/global-measles-vaccination-drive-protect-upto-45-million-children

Sommer, A., Tarwotjo, I., Djunaedi, E., West, K. P., Jr, Loeden, A. A., Tilden, R., & Mele, L. (1986). Impact of vitamin A supplementation on childhood mortality. A randomized controlled community trial. *Lancet, 1*(8491), 1169–1173. https://doi.org/10.1016/s0140-6736(86)91157-8

Soucheray, S. (2019, November 1). Measles does long-term damage to immune system, studies show. Center for Infectious Disease Research and Policy. https://www.cidrap.umn.edu/news-perspective/2019/11/measles-does-long-term-damage-immune-system-studies-show

Starr, P. (2017). The social transformation of American medicine: The rise of a sovereign profession and the making of a vast industry. Basic Books. First edition 1982.

Steichen, O., & Dautheville, S. (2009). Koplik's spots in early measles. *CMAJ: Canadian Medical Association Journal, 180*(5), 583–584.

Stulpin, C. (2020, February 13). US measles outbreaks cost $42 million, according to "conservative" estimate. Healio. https://www.healio.com/news/infectious-disease/20200213/us-measles-outbreaks-cost-42-million-according-to-conservative-estimate

Sudfeld, C. R., Navar, A. M., & Halsey, N. A. (2010, April 1). Effectiveness of measles vaccination and vitamin A treatment. *International Journal of Epidemiology, 39*(1), 48–55. https://doi.org.10.1093/ije/dyq021

Taylor, L., Swerdfeger, A., & Eslick, G. (2014). Vaccines are not associated with autism: An evidence-based meta-analysis of case-control and cohort studies. *Science Direct, 32*(29), 3623–3629. http://dx.doi.org/10.1016/j.vaccine.2014.04.085

Trentini, F., Poletti, P., Melegaro, A., & Merler, S. (2019, May 17). The introduction of "no jab, no school" policy and the refinement of measles immunisation strategies in high-income countries. *BMC Medicine, 17*(86). https://doi.org/10.1186/s12916-019-1318-5

U.S. National Library of Medicine. (n.d.). *ClinicalTrials.gov*. https://clinicaltrials.gov/

Wellcome. (2020). Wellcome trust survey. Chapter 5: Attitudes to vaccines. https://wellcome.org/reports/wellcome-global-monitor/2018/chapter-5-attitudes-vaccines

World Health Organization. (2021). Immunization, vaccines, and biological: WHO recommended surveillance standard of measles.

World Health Organization. (2020, November 12). Worldwide measles deaths climb 50% from 2016 to 2019 claiming over 207,500. https://www.who.int/news/item/12-11-2020-worldwide-measles-deaths-climb-50-from-2016-to-2019-claiming-over-207-500-lives-in-2019

World Health Organization. (2018–2019). How Romania's evidence-based communication and vaccination catch-up campaign led to better coverage among vulnerable groups. https://open.who.int/2018-19/country/ROU

World Health Organization, Regional Office for Africa. (2019). Measles. https://www.afro.who.int/health-topics/measles

Yang, H. M., Mao, M., & Wan, C. (2005). Vitamin A for treating measles in children. *Cochrane Database of Systematic Reviews, 2005*(4), 1479. https://doi.org/10.1002/14651858.CD001479.pub3

Yang, Q., Chuanxi, F., Wang, N., Dong, Z., Hu, W., & Wang, M. (2014). The effects of weather conditions on measles incidence in Guangzhou, Southern China. *Human Vaccines & Immunotherapeutics, 10*(4), 1104–1110. https://doi.org/10.4161/hv.27826

Index

About the Author

Dr. Patricia Clayton-LeVasseur has been in nursing practice for over twenty years. She has an extensive background in critical care, neuroscience, and education. She received her philosophy in nursing degree from Barry University. Currently, she is an associate professor at AdventHealth University. Dr. Clayton-LeVasseur is a member of the American Association of Neuroscience Nurses and the National League for Nursing. She has published articles in peer-reviewed nursing journals and presented at several international nursing conferences.